The Sleep Habits of

Sleep Habits

JOURNAL

*Practices, Prayers, and Devotions
to Ease Your Sleepless Nights*

BENJAMIN LONG, MD

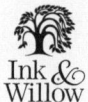

Ink &
Willow

Ink & Willow
An imprint of the Penguin Random House Christian Publishing Group, a division of Penguin Random House LLC
1745 Broadway, New York, NY 10019
inkandwillow.com
penguinrandomhouse.com

An Ink & Willow Trade Paperback Original

Interior illustrations: shutterstock.com: **Alla Koala**, bed (page 79); **Amanita Silvicora**, person with phone (page 103); **Anastasiia Novikova**, earbuds (page 65); **Anatolir**, roller coasters (page 62); **Arfa Yudha**, rotary phone (page 155); **arum widyaningsih**, digital alarm clock (pages 34, 54, 64); **AspctStyle**, star icons (pages 5, 18, 30, 33, 54–55, 57, 69, 72–73, 75, 82, 96–97, 99, 109, 122–23, 125, 129, 151, 153, 166, 170–71); **creativestockpro**, pillows (page 72); **ekosuwandono**, clouds (pages 67–68) **FMStox**, traffic signs (pages 54, 150); **GoodStudio**, coffee cup and paper sheets (page 146); **Gorbash Varvara**, swirl pattern (pages 6, 43, 46, 84, 89, 111); **Dancake**, full moon with clouds (pages 2, 13, 36); **melonee**, signpost (pages 54, 96); **Pavlo S**, smartphone screen (page 65); **pingebat**, road (pages 54, 150); **Shafiq GFX**, star confetti (pages 154–55); **Studio_G**, dream cloud (page 78); **tan47**, luggage (pages 44–45); **Valedi**, moons and clouds (pages 19, 50–51, 114, 119, 122, 158–59); **VikiVector**, slide (page 63); **Yauheniya_Bandaruk**, clock (page 170)

Trade Paperback ISBN 978-0-593-60252-2
Ebook ISBN 978-0-593-60264-5

Printed in Malaysia

9 8 7 6 5 4 3 2 1

The authorized representative in the EU for product safety and compliance is Penguin Random House Ireland, Morrison Chambers, 32 Nassau Street, Dublin D02 YH68, Ireland. https://eu-contact.penguin.ie

BOOK TEAM: Editor: Leslie Calhoun • Production editor: Jessica Choi • Managing editor: Julia Wallace • Production manager: Linnea Knollmueller • Copy editor: Lisa Grimenstein • Proofreaders: Carrie Krause, Karissa Silvers

Book design by HANNAH HUNT and JESSIE KAYE
Cover design by ZAIAH ANTWI

Cover art: shutterstock.com: **galacticus,** night sky

For details on special quantity discounts for bulk purchases,
contact specialmarketscms@penguinrandomhouse.com.

Contents

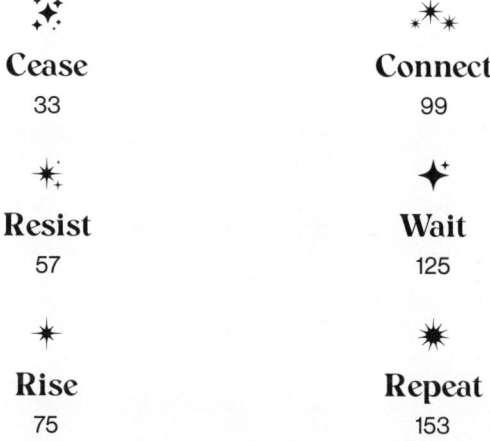

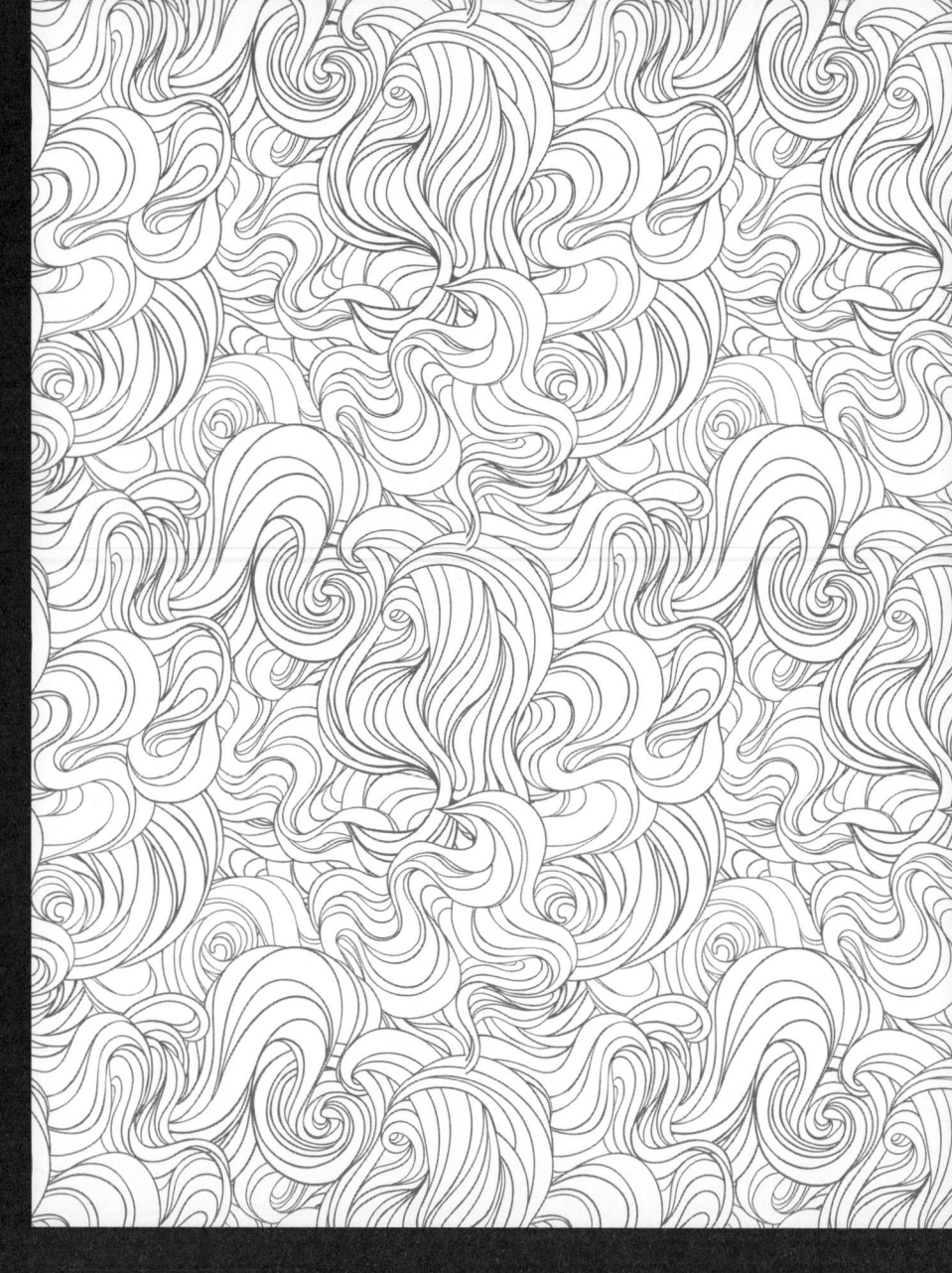

Introduction

SHIFTING THE SLEEPLESS NIGHT

When was your last sleepless night? Last night? Three years ago? Every night for the past three years? Benjamin Franklin once said, "In this world nothing can be said to be certain, except death and taxes,"* but I'd argue the sleepless night should go on that list too. Thankfully, the inevitability of these nights—whether a major struggle or minor annoyance—does not equal helplessness. In fact, from the moment you recognize it's time for bed throughout the next morning, you have dozens of opportunities to shift your experience.

This journal will help you explore these opportunities by providing lessons from medicine, theology, and the overlap between the two. From the medical world, I have included tips, activities, education, and supporting research. On the theological side, I have borrowed inspiration from one of the key ideas in the book *Theosomnia* by Rev. Dr. Andrew Bishop, which asserts that "Christian theology has a story to tell about sleep, drawing both from its texts and its practices."** This includes reflecting on concepts such as vulnerability, trust, and the motif of sleeplessness especially present in the Psalms.

─────────

*   NCC Staff, "Benjamin Franklin's Last Great Quote and the Constitution," National Constitution Center (blog), November 13, 2023, https://constitutioncenter.org/blog/benjamin-franklins-last-great-quote-and-the-constitution.

**   Andrew Bishop, *Theosomnia: A Christian Theology of Sleep* (London and Philadelphia: Jessica Kingsley Publishers, 2018), 14.

THE SLEEPLESS NIGHT RULES

Within the overlap between medicine and theology lies what I'm calling "The Sleepless Night Rules," which brings together a common, evidence-based intervention for insomnia and a Christian worldview. The rules are as follows:

1. **Cease** before bedtime and lie down once you feel sleepy.

2. **Rise** from bed if you cannot fall asleep.

3. **Connect** with God and **wait** to feel sleepy.

4. Lie down and **repeat** rules 2 and 3 if you cannot fall asleep.

5. **Resist** sleeping in and taking naps.

For those who have completed cognitive behavioral therapy for insomnia (CBT-I), these rules should look familiar. They are an adaptation of a classic component of CBT-I called *stimulus control therapy*. The original context behind the rules is to weaken any subconscious association between the bed or bedroom and being frustrated and awake. In adapting these rules, my hope is to direct your attention to not only your mind but also your spirit.

This journal is structured around the themes of the Sleepless Night Rules, though the observant reader may notice that the chapters of the journal are not in the same order as the rules themselves. (Kudos to all the people who just peeked ahead to confirm that's true!) This is intentional and reflects the order in which most people encounter their barriers. For example, "Cease" is chronologically first, but in the reading, "Resist" is next because those first few days are typically when you will most want to sleep in and nap!

HOW TO USE THIS JOURNAL

The journal begins with "My Sleep Journey," which will help you reflect on where you've been and how your sleep is going right now. The "Repeat" section at the end of the journal will prompt you to reflect on this section as well as on your overall growth during this sleep journey. You can complete the other sections consecutively or jump around depending on what you need in any given moment. The index may prove helpful in this regard, since it lists activities and practices by topic.

Within each section, you will find:

- **Professional Guidance:** Explore my advice, tips, and education on responding to sleeplessness with citations for any supporting research.

- **Biblical Perspective:** Reimagine your night from a Christian worldview with brief motivational devotions plus "Explore More" sections for digging deeper into selected passages.

- **Engaging Practices:** Complete activities that help calm your mind such as writing, drawing, and journaling, as well as Christian spiritual practices to encourage you to connect with God. You don't need to do every activity, but try to challenge yourself to consider ones that don't necessarily resonate with you.

- **Mile Markers:** Pause and reflect in the "Rest Areas" at the end of each section, where you can track your progress before moving on. Additionally, selected activities throughout the journal offer opportunities to gauge progress from previous sections. These will be noted as "Mile Markers," which will let you know that the particular activity is dependent upon completion of a previous page.

THEOSOMNIA

Ultimately, the goal of this journal is not to optimize or "biohack" your sleep. Nor is it necessarily to improve your sleep (although this will likely happen). Rather, the goal is to bring your sleep before God. It is transformation into *theosomnia*. Coined by Dr. Bishop, *theosomnia* literally means "'God-sleep' . . . hallowed sleep: in other words, sleep that is intentionally open to God; is blessed by God; and is offered to God.'" Bishop writes:

> ***Theosomnia*** is the sleep of the disciple drawn from the sleep seen in Jesus as he slept in the boat on the Sea of Galilee during the storm (Mark 4.35–41 and parallels). This is sleep of radical openness to the Father, since it is a Christological posture. Theosomnia acknowledges that sleep is a time when God can work deep within the self, when control is lost and the ego, like the storm, is stilled: "He must increase, but I must decrease" (John 3.30).**

May this journal help restore some peace to your bedtime routines. As you journey through its pages, my hope is that you will discover more rest, comfort, and joy despite your sleepless nights.

---

*   Bishop, *Theosomnia*, 24.

**   Bishop, 24.

Disclaimer

This book does not constitute a therapeutic relationship with the author. This resource is not intended as a substitute for professional medical advice, diagnosis, or treatment. Always seek the advice of your physician or other qualified health professional with any questions you may have regarding a medical condition. Never disregard professional medical advice or delay in seeking it because of something you have read in this book.

Unfortunately, not everyone has equal access to healthcare, and the demand for sleep health support often outpaces the number of qualified professionals to meet it. Despite this, the following groups should discuss the Sleepless Night Rules with a qualified health professional prior to implementing them: persons with limited mobility that restricts their ability to get out of bed safely and persons with a diagnosis that is exacerbated by temporary poor sleep (e.g., schizophrenia, bipolar disorder, or seizures). For these individuals, this resource will still be helpful, but the safest option would be to work with a health professional who can adjust the Sleepless Night Rules to meet your specific needs. Additionally, for persons with PTSD, panic attacks, or trauma that is associated with the bedroom, please note that this journal is not designed to specifically address those issues. As such, some of the practices and activities may be triggering. In those cases, I would recommend completing this journal in collaboration with a mental health professional who has experience in dealing with trauma to further support your mental health needs.

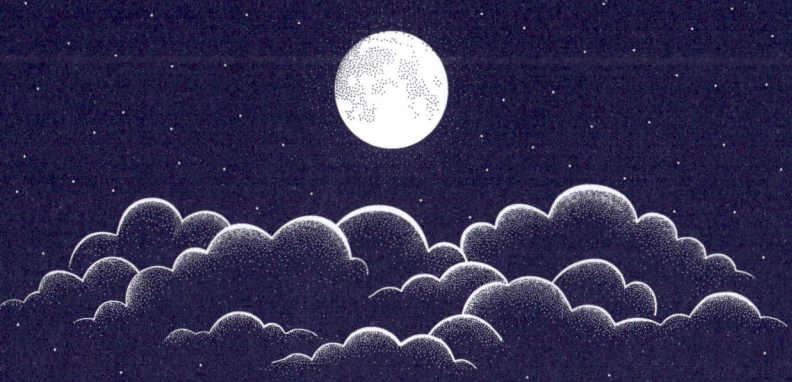

My Sleep Journey

To see and fully appreciate the impact of your journey,
it's important to have a clear picture of what came before.
Since the story of your sleepless night probably did not
start yesterday, this section offers space to reflect on
your past and current experience of sleeplessness.

My Sleep History

Reflect on your sleep as a child and write down any memories that come to mind. These can be happy, sad, or anything in between.

When did your difficulty with sleep begin? What was happening in your life around that time?

_____

_____

_____

_____

_____

_____

How have your challenges with sleep progressed (i.e., have they gotten better, stayed the same, or gotten worse, or are they on and off)?

_____

_____

_____

_____

_____

_____

_____

What has happened in your life since the beginning of your sleep problems?

_____

_____

_____

_____

_____

_____

_____

_____

_____

_____

_____

_____

_____

_____

_____

_____

_____

_____

How Insomnia Works

Insomnia develops when a precipitating event pushes you above the insomnia threshold. Even if the impact of the event improves, insomnia can continue if you adopt maladaptive factors in response to your insomnia. These factors can be personal or environmental and triggered by new events or your own decisions. The three main categories are:

Predisposing Factors

- family history of insomnia
- anxious personality
- hyperarousal (i.e., easily on "high alert")
- advancing age
- female
- socioeconomic status
- community violence

Precipitating Factors

- new diagnosis/illness
- stressful life events (e.g., death, deadlines, job loss, experience of abuse/violence)
- change in your social environment (e.g., moving, getting married, having a newborn/adopting a child)

Perpetuating Factors

- increasing time in bed (i.e., sleeping in or napping)
- tossing and turning all night
- doing more non-sleep-related activities (e.g., studying, working, scrolling on your phone) in your bedroom
- avoiding or ignoring your precipitating factors

After reviewing the list of insomnia factors, fill in the bars with your barriers to good sleep.

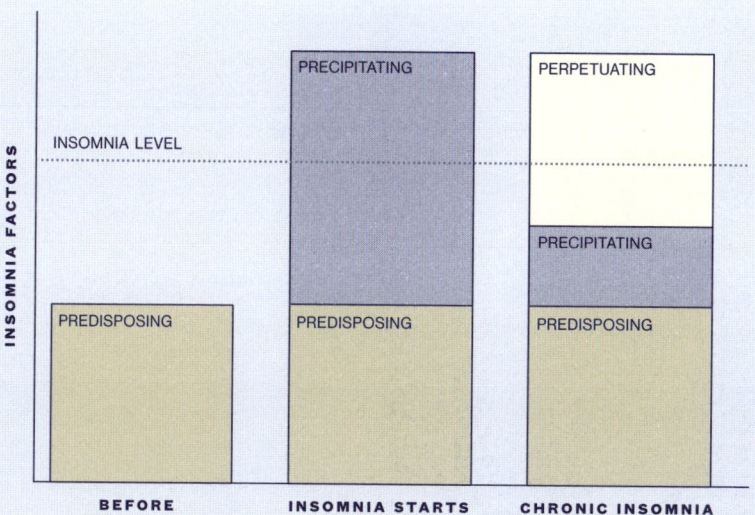

My Typical Night

Jot down some notes about your typical night hour by hour, including what you are thinking and feeling along the way. If it is difficult for you to remember how you feel at certain parts of the night, take one to two nights to observe what you're thinking and feeling in real time. It's okay if you don't have something to note for every hour. You might only record your thoughts and feelings for the first part of the night, the middle, or the early hours of the morning.

TIME	ACTIONS	THOUGHTS AND FEELINGS
6:00 P.M.		
7:00 P.M.		
8:00 P.M.		
9:00 P.M.	Brush teeth	Deadline next week
10:00 P.M.		I need to buy groceries tomorrow.
11:00 P.M.		
12:00 A.M.		Am I doing enough?

TIME	ACTIONS	THOUGHTS AND FEELINGS
1:00 A.M.	Toss and turn	Frustrated my mind won't turn off
2:00 A.M.		
3:00 A.M.		
4:00 A.M.		
5:00 A.M.		
6:00 A.M.	Wake up	
7:00 A.M.		
8:00 A.M.		

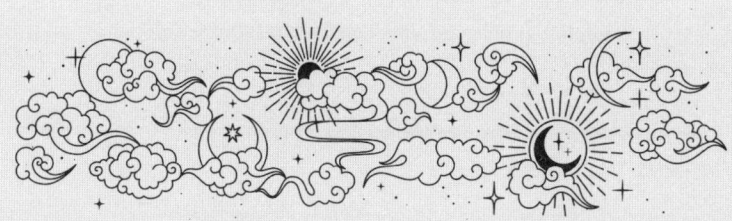

The Mind of Christ

> One of those days Jesus went out to a mountainside
> to pray, and spent the night praying to God.
>
> —Luke 6:12, NIV

As believers, our goal should be formation into Christ, or as mentioned in the New Testament, formation into the "mind of Christ" (see 1 Corinthians 2:16; Philippians 2:5; and Romans 12:2). While Jesus's teachings are an excellent entry point into His mind, we should also consider His actions. For example, how did He live His daily life? More specifically for our purposes in this book, how did He spend His *nights*?

According to several of the Gospels, Jesus often connected with God during the night (see Matthew 14:23 and Mark 14:32–41). Verses like these have inspired a rich tradition of nighttime prayers and forgoing sleep. But before you set off to pray on the nearest mountain, remember that you are not a "first-century, celibate Jewish rabbi," living in ancient Judea.[*] John Mark Comer puts it this way:

> It's a bit hard to ask [what would Jesus do?] if your current work is raising a two-year-old or teaching kindergarten or writing software or designing the HVAC system for a new building downtown—much less doing any of the latter *while* raising your two-year-old. Instead, ask this: How would Jesus live if he had my gender, place, personality profile, age, life stage, job, resources, and address?[**]

---

[*]   John Mark Comer, *Practicing the Way* (New York: WaterBrook, 2024), 123.

[**]   Comer, 123.

This question applies to your sleep journey as well. That is, how would Jesus walk through *your* sleepless night if He were you? Would He respond in anger or frustration at Himself? Would He be irritable with others the next morning because of fatigue? Would He start dreading the coming of night?

Scripture may not give us examples of Jesus struggling to fall asleep, but it does offer stories of trying circumstances. In those situations — when He faced impatient crowds, argumentative religious leaders, or dangerous politicians — how did He respond?

What do you think you can learn from Jesus's responses to frustrating situations, and how might you be able to apply that to your own sleepless nights?

_____

_____

_____

_____

_____

_____

_____

_____

_____

_____

_____

Light and Sight

Ask [the Holy Spirit] for light and sight that you may attain a perfect knowledge of yourself. . . . Knowledge of our spiritual progress depends on examination of this kind.

–Francis de Sales[*]

Recall your most recent sleepless night. Without judging yourself or your experience, invite the Holy Spirit to guide you through each moment. As you bring these memories to the present, explore at what moments you feel closer to God or farther away. Are you becoming a person of love, joy, peace, patience, kindness, goodness, faithfulness, gentleness, and self-control—or something else? Your answer will become a baseline for you to reflect on as you progress in your sleep journey.

End this practice with prayer, and as you consider your typical night, ask God to give you a word or phrase to describe who you are being formed into. Write down any words or phrases from your prayer time. If nothing comes, that's okay. Keep returning and asking.

_____

_____

_____

_____

_____

_____

[*] Brant Pitre, *Introduction to the Spiritual Life: Walking the Path of Prayer with Jesus* (New York: Image, 2021), 205.

Hope

We expect certain things out of sleep. When we are at a roadblock, we "sleep on it," hoping for a solution in the morning. When exhausted from the stress of the day, we hope for a "good night's rest."

People without disordered sleep typically rely on sleep intuitively, but for someone living on four to six hours of nightly sleep, those extra few hours can be elusive. The missed benefits of sleep can fuel a longing in one's heart. But know this: You don't need eight hours of sleep to flourish. Insomnia may be a barrier to navigate, but flourishing and living with insomnia are not mutually exclusive. Sometimes the first step to overcoming your barrier is simply to confront your expectations of it.

So, what would be different for you if you *could* get more sleep? What would change in your life?

If I could get seven to nine hours of sleep, then _____

_____

_____

_____

_____

_____

_____

_____

_____

_____

_____

Delight in the Night

Blessed is the one
> who does not walk in step with the wicked
or stand in the way that sinners take
> or sit in the company of mockers,
but whose delight is in the law of the Lord,
> and who meditates on his law day and night.

—PSALM 1:1–2, NIV

When you hear the phrase "day and night," what comes to mind? Many might interpret it as "a lot" or "all the time." Is there a difference between that and "day and night"? Does the verse affect us differently if we say "who meditates on his law [all the time]"?

Many people go to bed without praying, and far fewer engage in prayer or Bible reading when they find themselves unable to sleep. Of course, most people aren't *actively* avoiding these activities. They just don't think to do them! We are too easily habituated to filling our time with entertainment, distraction, or productivity. But if we want to be formed into the image of Christ, one of the first steps is to find pathways to connect with God, even in our sleepless nights.

At the end of a chaotic day, the idea of doing something different from your usual bedtime routine may feel overwhelming. But consider what Psalm 1 says about the person who is blessed, or "happy" (NRSVA). They are like a tree planted by a source of water that keeps its leaves from withering. Roots take time to grow, and change does not happen overnight; but the more you root yourself in God, the more comfort you will discover in His teachings.

How can you prioritize time to delight in God's Word? Do you have a favorite verse or one you find especially comforting? Write it down in the space below.

_____

_____

_____

_____

_____

_____

_____

_____

_____

_____

_____

_____

_____

_____

_____

_____

Explore More

Read through Psalm 1 and note the contrast between the "blessed" and the "wicked." Fill in the columns below with the attributes and actions specific to each.

BLESSED	WICKED

Practicing Gratitude

While gratitude alone will not fix your sleep problems, it does offer an important connection between sleep quality and spiritual well-being.*

Write down three things for which you are thankful:

1. _____

2. _____

3. _____

*   Paul J. Mills et al., "The Role of Gratitude in Spiritual Well-Being in Asymptomatic Heart Failure Patients," *Spirituality in Clinical Practice (Washington, D.C.)* 2, no. 1 (March 2015): 5–17, https://doi .org/10.1037/scp0000050.

Ordered Creation

God called the light "day," and the darkness he
called "night." And there was evening, and there
was morning—the first day.

—Genesis 1:5, **NIV**

God placed a rhythmic order into creation. Night and day, evening and
morning, season after season, year after year. The biblical authors were in
tune with these cyclical patterns.

However, modernity—with its innovations and advances—distances us
from these patterns. Cellphones, TV screens, and lightbulbs blur daily rhythms.
The economic pressure for twenty-four-hour productivity in most Western
countries demands exertion that is often at odds with human limitations. In
general, sleep in Western-educated, industrialized, wealthy, and democratic
societies is influenced by a mindset of independence and regimented control.
But sleep in an ancient, Near-Eastern context held no illusion of control. Imagine
no internet or electricity. Night so black you couldn't see your hand in front
of your face. Noises emerging from the darkness might have caused you to
wonder whether you would make it through the night at all. But then morning
would come. Rest followed by work. You would lie down and then rise. You
would sleep and—for much of human history—hope to wake with the sunrise.

This pattern of ordered daily life is prominent in the opening verses of
the Bible. God brings order out of "a formless and desolate emptiness"
(Genesis 1:2, **NASB**), and each day He adds more to His growing creation.
In between each day of creation is the recurring phrase "there was
evening and there was morning." Where there was once chaos, God spoke
a certain, cyclical order into existence.

Sleep is part of that ordered creation. No matter how chaotic or
disconnected the world may seem, all waking ultimately gives way to
sleep. The rhythm of God's creation is in and around us.

How does it make you feel to know that all waking—and sleeplessness—
will eventually be followed by sleeping?

_____

_____

_____

_____

_____

_____

_____

_____

_____

_____

_____

_____

_____

_____

_____

_____

_____

_____

_____

Rest Area

Before going further on this journey, calculate your average daily sleep (including any naps). Doing this will provide an estimate of how much sleep you might need each night. Track your sleep for ten days and then figure out the average. If you're feeling overwhelmed, you can take a few nights or come back to this when you feel ready.

DAYS	HOURS
DAY 1	
DAY 2	
DAY 3	
DAY 4	
DAY 5	
DAY 6	
DAY 7	
DAY 8	
DAY 9	
DAY 10	
TOTAL	____ ÷ 10 = ____

Now answer the following questions:

When I lie down to sleep, I feel

_____

_____

_____

_____

_____

_____

It typically takes me _____ minutes/hours to fall asleep.

I sleep in or take a nap _____ days in a typical week.

The Sleepless Night
RULES

1. Cease before bedtime and lie
down once you feel sleepy.

2. Rise from bed if you
cannot fall asleep.

3. Connect with God and
wait to feel sleepy.

4. Lie down and repeat rules 2 and 3
if you cannot fall asleep.

5. Resist sleeping in and
taking naps.

So if we really intend to submit our bodies as living sacrifices to God, our first step well might be to start *getting enough sleep.*

—DALLAS WILLARD, *RENOVATION OF THE HEART*

Cease

*Cease before bedtime and lie
down once you feel sleepy.*

At the click of a button, your computer goes to sleep. But
have you ever considered how this level of technological
control might be influencing our expectations of human
sleep? Phrases like "recharge my batteries," "wind down
for the night," and "I just can't turn off my mind" reveal our
expectation for the mind and body to behave like a TV
responding to a remote. But we are not machines. We
need time.

    This brings us to the problem of ceasing (or, really, the
lack thereof). Whether it's one more TV show, one more email,
or one more chapter, we often find it difficult to maintain a
consistent transition to bedtime. This section explores the
time that occurs between us starting to think about bedtime
and our heads actually hitting the pillow. Ceasing is hard and
countercultural, but God invites us to embrace our limitations
and practice trust by choosing to stop the activity of the day
and willingly enter rest.

My Bedtime Goal

For many of us, bedtime is a range: We may say it's between 8:30 and 9:30 or even 10:30 and midnight. Tasks, responsibilities, or the reprieve from them often contribute to the variability. But the root problem is not unpredictability. It's typically due to a lack of planning. Just because you don't have a remote to turn off the chaos of life doesn't mean that setting a specific bedtime is impossible. On the contrary, you may be surprised just how easy it is and how much it can help.

If you struggle with a consistent bedtime, commit to a specific hour and minute for transitioning to bed just for this week.

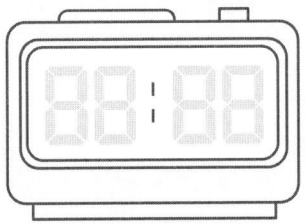

Healthy Bedtime Habits

- **Set an alarm for bedtime.** This is your line in the sand to cease from work, worrying, and screens. It's not when you plan to be *in* bed, but rather when you transition to your bedroom. Try to give yourself a minimum of thirty minutes before "lights out."

- **Turn off the lights.** This is one of the most important and least followed sleep habits: Turn off your lights thirty to sixty minutes before bedtime. If you are having difficulty maintaining a specific bedtime, schedule a time to turn everything off. The strongest cue for your body's circadian rhythm is light—and not just from your phone, but from the lights in your home as well. If turning off the lights seems unrealistic, try installing dimmable lights or buying plug-in nightlights to place around your home.

- **Put your screens to bed.** As John Mark Comer writes, "Parent your phone."[*] Many apps are designed to keep you engaged for as long as possible and can impact your sleep.[**] So choosing *when* to put the screens away will help with your transition to bedtime. Instead of using screens right up until bedtime, turn them off at least thirty minutes before heading to bed. If you are doing assignments for night school or finishing work (and cannot finish in the morning), wear blue-light-blocking glasses.[***]

---

[*]   John Mark Comer, *The Ruthless Elimination of Hurry* (New York: WaterBrook, 2019), 227.

[**]   Liese Exelmans and Jan Van den Bulck, "Bedtime Mobile Phone Use and Sleep in Adults," *Social Science & Medicine* 148 (2016): 93–101, https://doi.org/10.1016/j.socscimed.2015.11.037.

[***]   Karolina Janků et al., "Block the Light and Sleep Well: Evening Blue Light Filtration as a Part of Cognitive Behavioral Therapy for Insomnia," *Chronobiology International* 37, no. 2 (2020): 248–59, https://doi.org/10.1080/074205 28.2019.1692859. A systematic review (https://doi.org/10.1093/sleepadvances/zpaa002) has found mixed results (neutral to positive), so it's worth a shot.

- **Set the remote down.** Before bed, choose an activity you enjoy but find easy to transition away from (i.e., don't watch that suspenseful drama series that always ends on a cliffhanger). Bingeable shows are not only difficult to turn off but also directly detrimental to calming your mind, since consuming emotional content before bed has been shown to affect your sleep as well.*

- **Ask for help.** Whether you're parenting a newborn, training a new puppy, or just trying to survive a busy, sleep-deprived season of life, ask for help! You may be surprised by how many people are willing to hold the baby, walk the dog, or even help out around the house so you can catch up on some sleep.

* Suresh C. Joshi, Jay Woodward, and Steven Woltering, "Nighttime Cell Phone Use and Sleep Quality in Young Adults," *Sleep and Biological Rhythms* 20 (November 2021): 97–106, https://doi.org/10.1007/s41105-021-00345-6.

My Sleep Habit

Write down a sleep habit you can commit to in the upcoming week, whether that's going to bed at a specific time, turning off the lights, putting away your devices, or something else.

Sleep as Surrender

But you, **Lord,** are a shield around me,
     my glory, the One who lifts my head high.
I call out to the **Lord,**
     and he answers me from his holy mountain.

I lie down and sleep;
     I wake again, because the **Lord** sustains me.

                       –Psalm 3:3–5, **NIV**

Do you ever think of sleep as a barrier to productivity?

Being hesitant about sleep is certainly not a modern phenomenon. Clement of Alexandria, a second-century church father, wrote, "For the oppression of sleep is like death, which forces us into insensibility . . . and all of us should, so to speak, fight against sleep, accustoming ourselves to this gently and gradually, so that through wakefulness we may partake of life for a longer period."* To be clear, Clement was not necessarily anti-sleep; he was primarily cautioning against excessive and indulgent sleep. But this idea still strikes a chord for modern audiences: Sleep feels like a waste of time.

Don't get me wrong. Many of us love sleeping. But even though we enjoy the benefits of sleep, spending a third of our lives motionless in bed can feel unproductive. However, maybe the extent of time spent in this vulnerable state says something quite profound.

Dallas Willard writes that the body "*must* be weaned away from its tendencies to always take control, to run the world, to achieve and produce, to attain gratification. These are its habitual tendencies learned

---

* Clement of Alexandria, *The Writings of Clement of Alexandria,* trans. Rev. William Wilson, Book II, Chapter IX, "On Sleep" (Edinburgh: T & T Clark, 1867), 242–43.

in a fallen world.'"* In other words, our constant drive to *do* is something we must unlearn.

Psalm 3 reveals a creative response to our natural tendencies and the oppressive restriction we face. Instead of always being on the go, we can embody trust by ceasing activity for sleep. Ceasing acknowledges our vulnerability while preaching the power of God. One commentator writes, "We live in a world where verbal, psychological, and even physical abuse seem to be commonplace. . . . The result of having our spirit violated by those we trust is more than anger; often our sense of self is undermined as well. . . . We can be too easily persuaded that the enemy's line is right: 'God will not deliver you.'"** And yet each morning we wake is a testament of God's sustaining power. We can cease because God has everything under control—even without our help.

How firmly do you trust that God will deliver you from sleeplessness or other challenges you are facing? What lies of the enemy might be keeping you from sleep?

_____

_____

_____

_____

_____

_____

---

* Dallas Willard, *Renovation of the Heart: Putting on the Character of Christ* (Colorado Springs: NavPress, 2021), 182.

** Gerald Henry Wilson, *The NIV Application Commentary: Psalms Volume 1* (Grand Rapids, Mich.: Zondervan, 2002), 137.

Explore More

Read Psalm 3 a few times.

Try to imagine yourself as the psalmist. King David wrote this psalm when he was fleeing Jerusalem—literally running for his life—to evade his son Absalom (see 2 Samuel 15–16). As you go through the psalm, pause at each *Selah* and reflect on the section you've just read. Note any thoughts or takeaways.

Verses 1–2: _____

Verses 3–4: _____

Verses 5–8: _____

Trace how the description of the enemy builds. The word often translated as "many" is "a verb meaning 'have become many, have multiplied.'" This situation is not "a static circumstance of oppression but a dangerously escalating situation that threatens imminently to consume the psalmist."* List all the descriptions of the adversary.

- _____
- _____
- _____
- _____
- _____

In verse 2, the mocking words of the enemy are "intended to shake him to the very roots—to leave him naked and vulnerable to their attack."** The original Hebrew word for "deliverance" connotes "removing restriction

---

*   Wilson, 129.

**   Wilson, 129.

and providing room."* This definition adds to the swelling sense of danger, since the psalmist finds himself in a situation where he wants "room, space to breathe, [to] maneuver, perhaps even escape," but that is precisely "what the opponents intend to deny."** Can you relate to this?

Now list David's description of God in verses 3–4 (on page 38):

- He describes the Lord as a _____
- His _____
- The One who _____
- He _____

Danger may be approaching, but what does David's reply demonstrate?

_____

David's understanding of God's faithfulness supports his unexpected response in verse 5. In the face of enemies that have "set themselves against [him] all around," David is able to lie down and sleep. How crazy is that? The enemy is oppressive and threatening, yet instead of running or fighting, David *ceases*. He is then able to express gratitude in the final verses due to the refreshing confidence that comes after a good night's sleep.

How has God sustained you and delivered you from opposition in your life?

_____

_____

_____

===

*   Wilson, 129.

**   Wilson, 130.

Practicing Gratitude

Ceasing acknowledges your lack of control. It is easy to convince yourself that things will fall apart without your efforts. But God holds all creation together. From far-off galaxies to your beating heart, there is a lot to be thankful for that God is in control of.

Write down three things you're thankful that God holds together:

1. _____

2. _____

3. _____

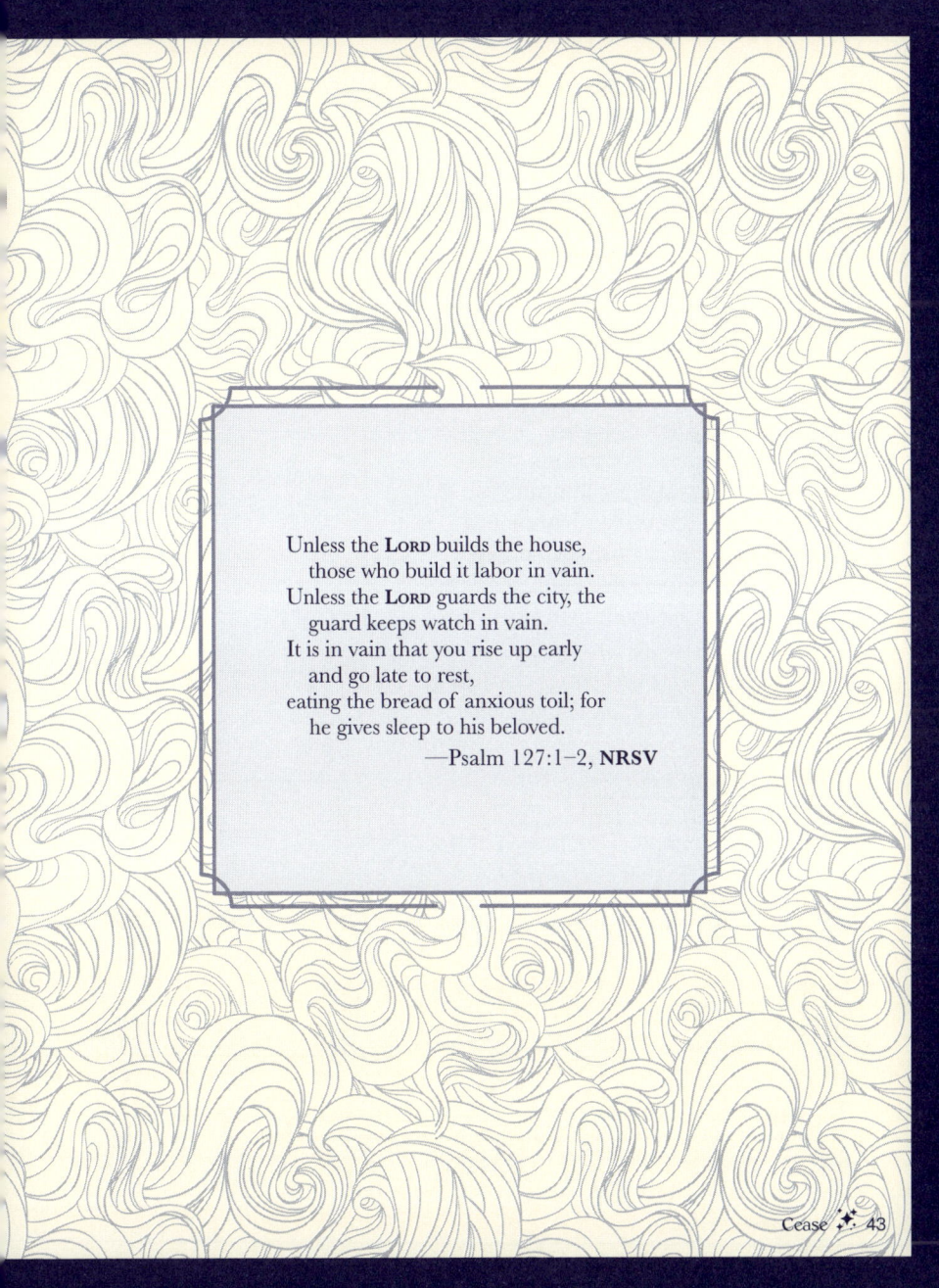

Unless the **Lord** builds the house,
	those who build it labor in vain.
Unless the **Lord** guards the city, the
	guard keeps watch in vain.
It is in vain that you rise up early
	and go late to rest,
eating the bread of anxious toil; for
	he gives sleep to his beloved.

—Psalm 127:1–2, **NRSV**

Unpack the List

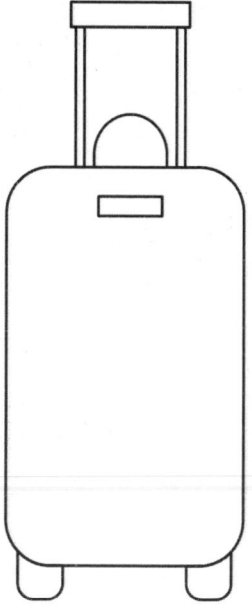

Do you have a difficult time "turning off" your mind to fall asleep?

Write down the things on your mind: the to-do lists, the worries, and anything else taking up thought space. By putting pen to page, you'll find that it is often easier to let go of those thoughts.* I recommend completing this practice before your transition to bed and, if possible, not in your bed or bedroom. If you start to think about anything on the list after bedtime, try to remind yourself that it is written down and you don't have to concern yourself with it until later.

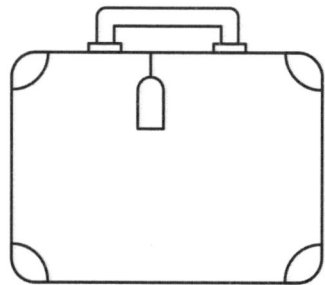

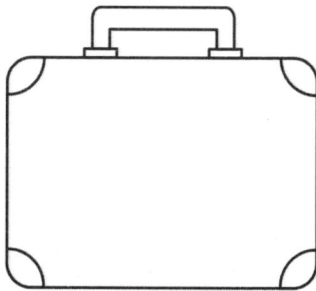

---

*   Michael K. Scullin et al., "The Effects of Bedtime Writing on Difficulty Falling Asleep: A Polysomnographic Study Comparing To-Do Lists and Completed Activity Lists," *Journal of Experimental Psychology* 147, no. 1 (2018): 139–46, https://doi.org/10.1037/xge0000374.

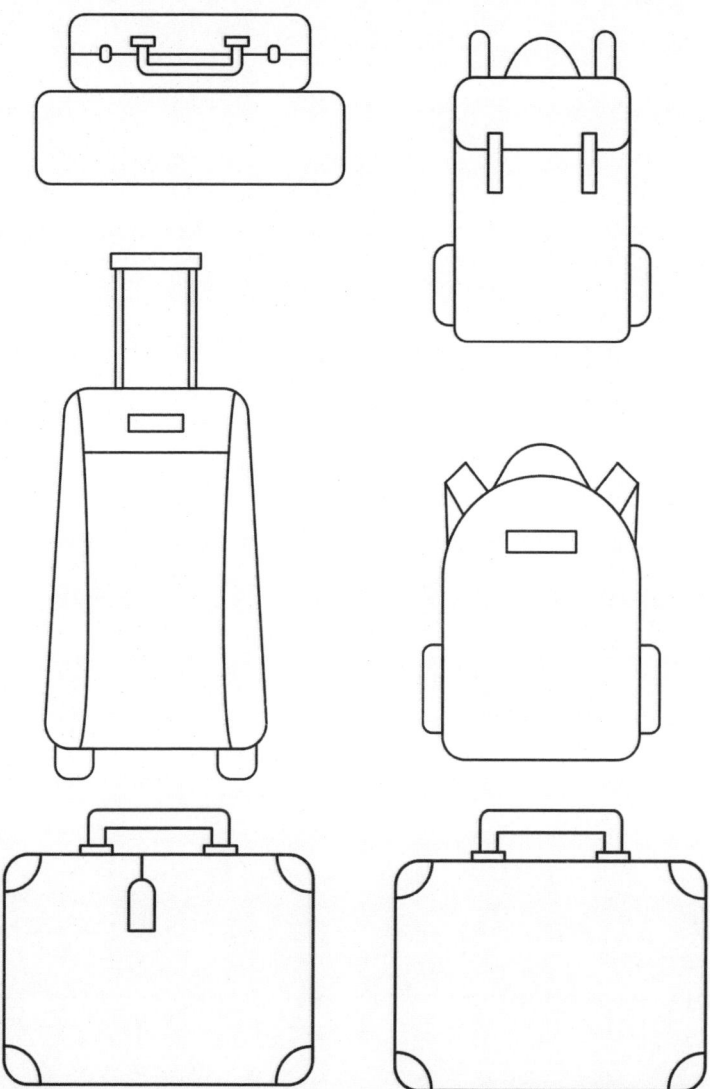

But I will give him the only gift he is still able to receive.... Sleep and be separated for some few hours from all the torments you have devised for yourself.

—C. S. LEWIS,
Aslan in *The Magician's Nephew*

The Examen

Attributed to Saint Ignatius of Loyola, the Daily Examen (or sometimes just called the Examen) is a contemplative practice that helps you to reflect on your day while inviting God to adjust the lens of your memory to illuminate the events or emotions you may have experienced. In practice, the Examen is a tool Christians can use to process their daily stress, practice gratitude, and discern God's presence and direction in their lives.

The Examen Practice

1. Settle into the moment with some deep breathing and shift your mind to become aware of God's presence.

2. Invite the Holy Spirit to reveal Himself and direct your time in prayer.

3. Once you've settled in, replay the events of your day with a posture of gratitude.

4. Allow your mind to linger, giving yourself grace to return to the moment when your thoughts wander.

5. Allow the Spirit to bring attention to people and circumstances you encountered throughout the day.

6. Look forward to tomorrow.

7. End your time in prayer in whatever way you feel led.

Remember Your Day

Take some time to journal about your day by responding to the prompts below or jotting down any moments as they come to you.

When did you experience peace, joy, or gratitude?

_____

_____

_____

_____

_____

_____

_____

When did you feel tension, either internally or externally?

_____

_____

_____

_____

_____

_____

_____

What else do you want to note about today?

_____

_____

_____

_____

_____

_____

_____

_____

_____

_____

_____

_____

_____

_____

_____

_____

_____

_____

_____

Draw the Sleepless Night

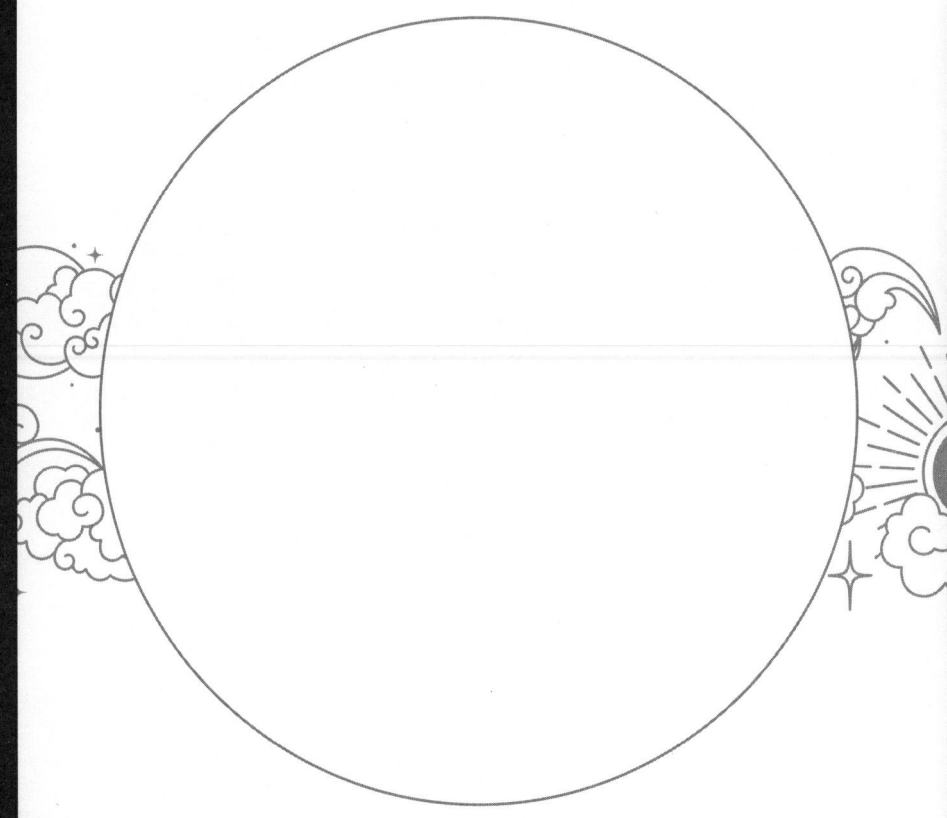

Use the following circles to draw how you feel about your sleepless nights.* Fill the circle with patterns, designs, colors, and/or a picture that represents your experience of a sleepless night. Try not to use any words.

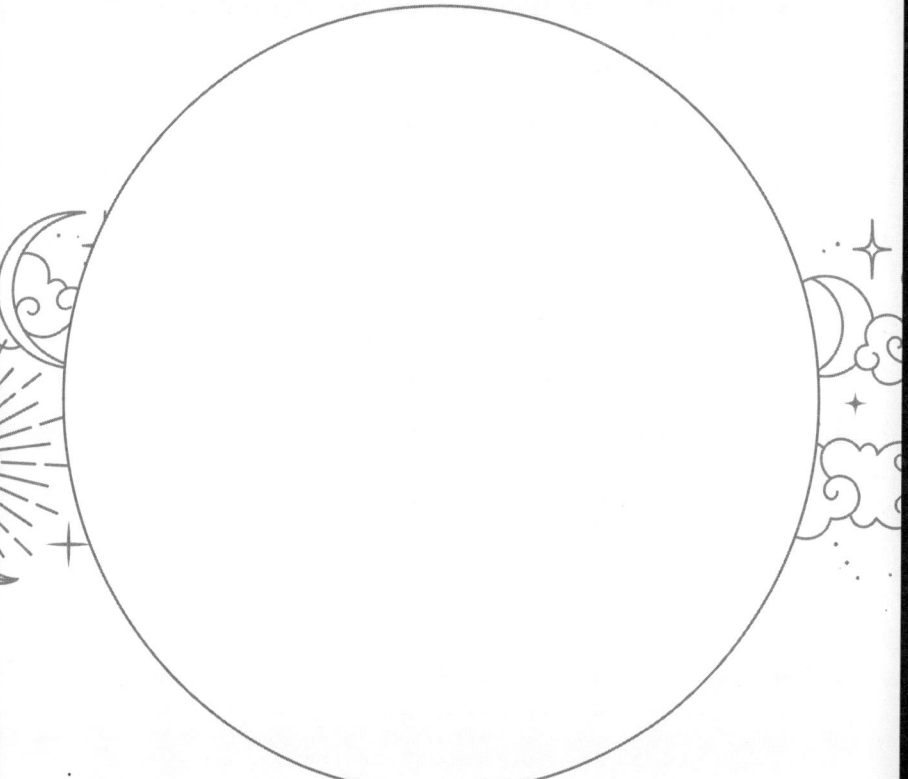

*   Wenny Ratnasari, Monty Satiadarma, and Roswiyani Roswiyani, "The Effect of Art Therapy Mandala to Reduce Symptoms of Depression in Adolescents with Insomnia," *International Journal of Application on Social Science and Humanities* 1, no. 1 (February 2023): 334–39, https://doi.org/10.24912/ijassh.v1i1.25814.

Memorizing Scripture

Choose one of the following verses to memorize and write it out in the space below. Meditate on this verse as you are transitioning to bedtime.

> I lie down and sleep;
>   I wake again, because the LORD sustains me.
> —Psalm 3:5, **NIV**

> Come to me, all you that are weary and are carrying heavy burdens, and I will give you rest. Take my yoke upon you, and learn from me; for I am gentle and humble in heart, and you will find rest for your souls. For my yoke is easy, and my burden is light.
> —Matthew 11:28–30, **NRSV**

_____

_____

_____

_____

_____

_____

_____

_____

_____

_____

A Prayer for Ceasing

To God-Who-Never-Sleeps,
we have too much to do,
and not enough time.
But You, Lord, rule over all creation—
even our to-do lists.
Remind us of our creatureliness and limitations,
which contrast with Your infinite love and provision.
Help us cease,
as an act of resistance,
against any idol of
productivity or prideful ambition.
Prepare our hearts to accept
Your gift of sleep tonight.

Write your own prayer of ceasing below:

_____

_____

_____

_____

_____

_____

_____

_____

_____

Rest Area

Commit to a consistent bedtime for one week and write that time on the clock below. Then shade in a stop sign for each night you're successful!

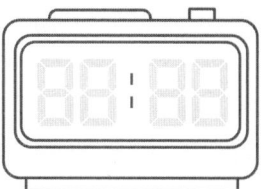

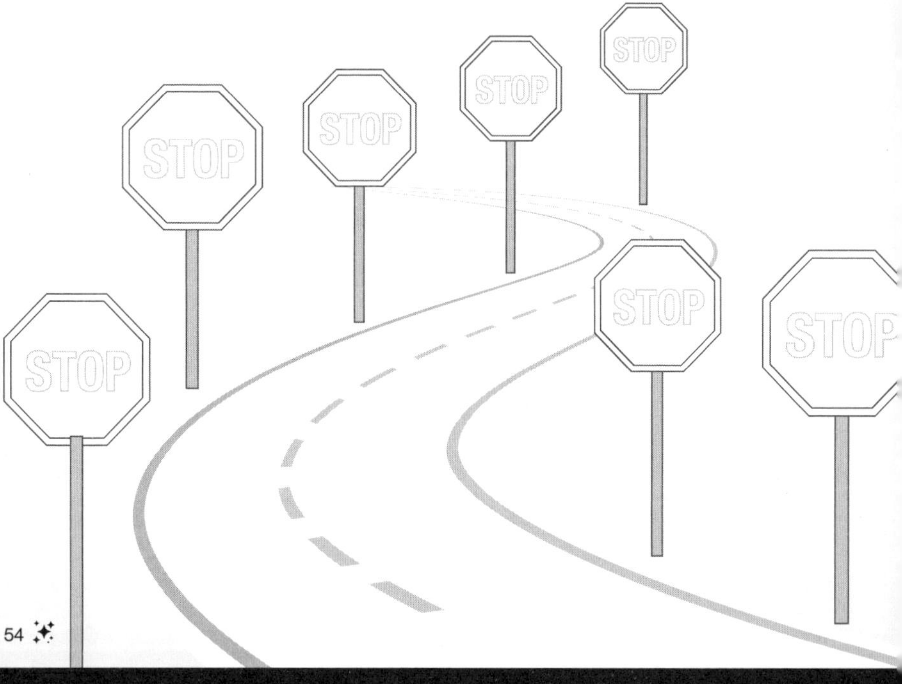

TRACKING YOUR
Sleep Journey

Just before getting into bed this week, track how you are feeling after ceasing from your day.

NIGHT 1	
NIGHT 2	
NIGHT 3	
NIGHT 4	
NIGHT 5	
NIGHT 6	
NIGHT 7	

Happiness is waking up, looking at the clock, and finding that you still have two hours left to sleep.

—ATTRIBUTED TO
CHARLES M. SCHULZ

Resist

*Resist sleeping in and
taking naps.*

A morning Jewish prayer offers fifteen blessings of gratitude
for the initial ordinary moments of the day. One of the fifteen
"gives thanks to God for removing 'sleep from the eyes,
slumber from the eyelids.'"* This line is thought to coincide
with the ordinary "moment when a person first washes his
face in the morning."**

  Similar to the one praying this prayer, you also have a
morning ritual. But instead of washing sleep from your eyes,
you may have a habit of hitting the snooze button, sleeping
in on weekends, or taking long naps. While these decisions
may feel good in the moment, they often have negative
consequences.

  In this section, we'll explore how to keep sleep in its place
and learn how to resist it.

---

* Charles Isbell, "Sleep from the Eyes, Slumber from the Eyelids," *Jewish Bible Quarterly* 34, no.
1 (2006): 39.

** Isbell, 39.

The Morning Routine

Shake off slumber from your eyelids with a morning routine that promotes wakefulness. Research has found that these activities lead to shorter and less severe sleep inertia:[*]

1. **Say no to snoozing.** Better yet, place your alarm on the other side of the room so you have to get out of bed to turn it off.

2. **Move your body.** Take a walk, do some chores, or just dance.

3. **Rinse with a splash of cold water.** Wash your hands or face, or take a full shower.

4. **Let in the light.** Send a strong wake-up signal to your brain through exposure to sunlight.

5. **Turn up the music.** Go to page 65 to create your get-up-and-go playlist.

6. **Talk to a friend.** Social interaction is a cue for your brain that it's time to be awake.

---

[*] Katherine Kaplan, David Talavera, and Allison Harvey, "Rise and Shine: A Treatment Experiment Testing a Morning Routine to Decrease Subjective Sleep Inertia in Insomnia and Bipolar Disorder," *Behaviour Research and Therapy* 111 (2018): 106–12, https://doi.org/10.1016/j.brat.2018.10.009.

Healthy Daytime Habits

- **Take short naps.** If you're struggling to resist sleep, take a ten- to fifteen-minute nap. A short nap can have the benefit of improving focus and mood without impacting your ability to fall asleep at night.

- **Anticipate your sleepiness.** Try to schedule activities that will help you stay awake for when you are the sleepiest during the day. You might call or talk to a friend, watch an engaging TV show, or work on a project or hobby that you find interesting.

- **Be intentional with your caffeine intake.** Caffeine is most effective if you consume it around thirty minutes before your expected decrease in alertness. It typically stays in your system for five to six hours. As such, the earlier in the day you can consume your caffeine, the better.

- **Get active.** Physical exertion sends a strong signal to your brain to stay awake. Additionally, strenuous exercise, as long as it is not within ninety minutes of falling asleep, may help you fall asleep quicker at night.[*] Plan ahead by writing down activities you can do to help you stay awake.

---

[*] D. J. Miller et al., "Moderate-Intensity Exercise Performed in the Evening Does Not Impair Sleep in Healthy Males," *European Journal of Sport Science* 20, no. 1 (2020): 80–89; Iuliana Hartescu, Kevin Morgan, and Clare Stevinson, "Increased Physical Activity Improves Sleep and Mood Outcomes in Inactive People with Insomnia: A Randomized Controlled Trial," *Journal of Sleep Research* 24, no. 5 (2015): 526–34.

Just a Little Sleep

A little sleep, a little slumber,
     a little folding of the hands to rest—
and poverty will come on you like a thief
     and scarcity like an armed man.

—Proverbs 6:10–11, **NIV**

Life in the ancient Near East included resting at midday (see Genesis 18:4 and 2 Samuel 4:5). However, that rest needed boundaries. Proverbs 6:9 sets the scene: "How long will you lie there, O lazybones? When will you rise from your sleep?" (**NRSVA**). The response with its thrice repeated "a little" emphasizes how innocuous these surrenders seem at the outset. Almost as if the person is saying, "I'm just closing my eyes for a minute. I'll fold my arms for a bit and *then* I'll be ready to work." But there is a reason the original Hebrew text refers to sleep and slumber in the plural. The author was emphasizing multiple "untimely instances of sleep."* The person in the proverb is not *intentionally* trying to forgo their work, but rather "deceives himself by the smallness of his surrenders. So, by inches and minutes, his opportunity slips away."** In other words, if you're not careful, sleep can intrude upon your day.

Does this mean you're doomed if you take a nap? Not necessarily. Rather, this is a cautionary tale of sleep's slow invasion. Later in Proverbs, the author explored the result of succumbing to these little sleeps. He passed by land "completely overgrown with thistles . . . covered with nettles, [with] its stone wall . . . broken down" (Proverbs 24:31, **NASB1995**).

Sleep is a gift, but without boundaries, it can have devastating consequences.

---

* Bruce Waltke, *The Book of Proverbs: Chapters 1–15* (Grand Rapids, Mich.: Wm. B. Eerdmans, 2004), 2497k. ProQuest Ebook Central.

** Derek Kidner, *Proverbs* (Downers Grove, Ill.: InterVarsity Press, 2018), 39.

How has your sleeping in or taking naps affected your daily
responsibilities?

_____

_____

_____

_____

_____

_____

_____

_____

_____

_____

_____

_____

_____

_____

_____

_____

_____

_____

_____

_____

Sleep Pressure
Roller Coaster

Imagine your sleepiness rising through the day like a roller coaster. The longer you're awake, the higher your sleep pressure builds. Taking a long nap steals from that pressure and makes it harder for you to fall asleep later.

Draw a stick figure on the ride you rode today.

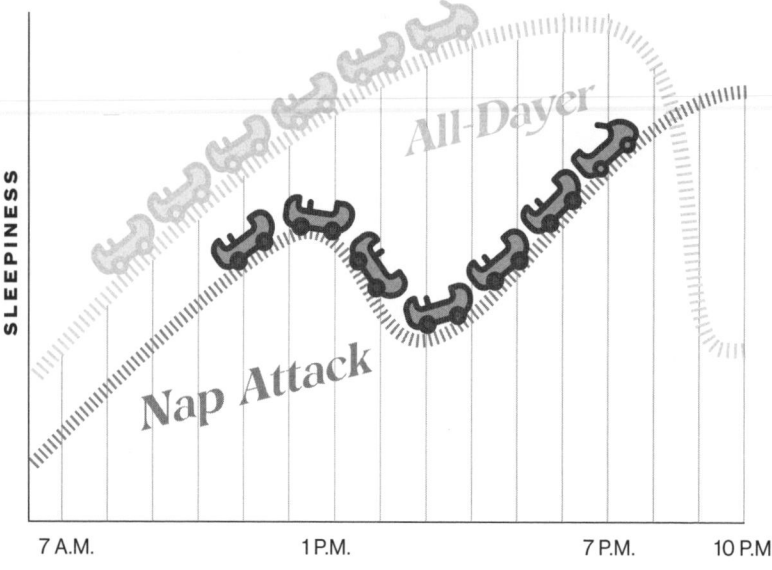

If you rode the "Nap Attack" today, no worries! You will find more rest when you hop on the "All-Dayer" tomorrow!

Your Circadian Slide

Draw a stick figure on the time when you feel sleepiest during the day.

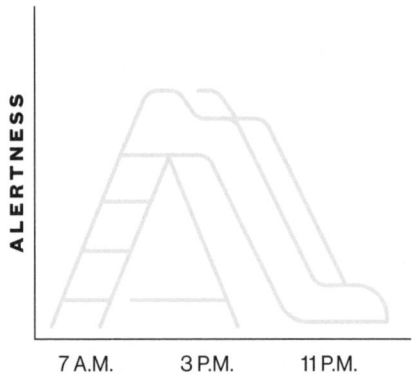

ALERTNESS

7 A.M.   3 P.M.   11 P.M.

     Everyone has a circadian rhythm (i.e., daily rhythm) that helps keep them awake. Most people's rhythm is on an upswing by midmorning and starts to plateau around lunchtime. This is why even after being awake for twenty-four hours, you'll notice a rise in energy the next morning. But the circadian rhythm also contributes to the "post-lunch slump" most people feel around two to four in the afternoon.

What time is your "post-lunch slump"?

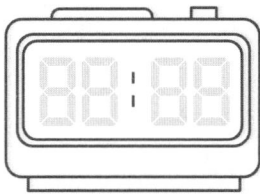

What can you do before the slump to not feel so sleepy?

_____

_____

_____

_____

_____

_____

_____

_____

_____

My Wake-Up Playlist

An energetic playlist can help wake you up in the morning or after a short nap.[*] Use the space below to create your own playlist of favorite "hype" songs.

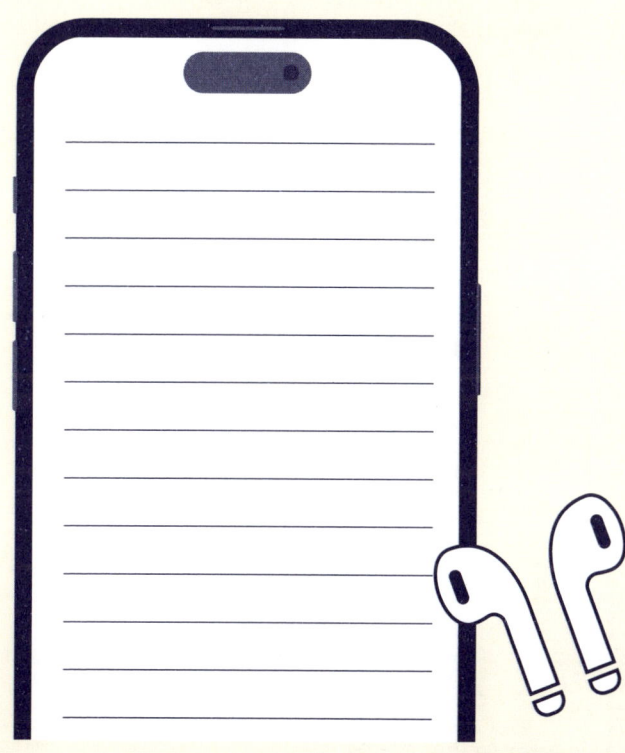

---

[*] Mitsuo Hayashi et al., "The Effects of the Preference for Music on Sleep Inertia After a Short Daytime Nap," *Sleep and Biological Rhythms* 2 (2004): 184–91.

Practicing Gratitude

Research suggests an "upward spiral between gratitude and joy."* Practicing gratitude paves the way to experiencing joy, which in turn makes you inclined to be more grateful. So make a habit of counting your blessings. List several here:

1. _____

2. _____

3. _____

4. _____

5. _____

* Philip C. Watkins et al., "Joy Is a Distinct Positive Emotion: Assessment of Joy and Relationship to Gratitude and Well-Being," *The Journal of Positive Psychology* 13, no. 5 (2018): 522–39.

Savor God's Creation

Repeatedly in Genesis 1, God looks at creation and calls it good. When was the last time you did the same?

Take a twenty-minute walk for the sole purpose of observing as many sights, sounds, smells, and other sensations within God's good creation. As you notice something, let it linger in your mind and give thanks for it. When you savor something, you build gratitude in the present, which then brings you more joy and peace. In fact, the practice of savoring has been shown to increase happiness after one week of implementing.[*]

How do you feel after savoring? Reflect on your experience below.

_____

_____

_____

_____

_____

_____

_____

_____

_____

_____

[*] Fred B. Bryant and Joseph Veroff, *Savoring: A New Model of Positive Experience* (Mahwah, N.J.: Lawrence Erlbaum Associates, 2007).

A Prayer for Resisting

Lord Jesus Christ,
I ache for rest.
It is time to wake and work,
but exhaustion hangs over me.
I don't know how to get through this day.
Grant me Your presence, wisdom, and the strength to resist.
Remove the sleep from my eyes and slumber from my eyelids,
so that I may see the work You have for me today,
and the gift of sleep You hold for me tonight.

Write your own prayer to help you resist sleeping in and taking naps.

_____

_____

_____

_____

_____

_____

_____

_____

_____

_____

Pivot

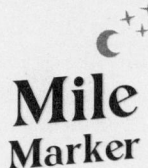

Mile
Marker

Are you noticing a change in how you feel about the night? Find the word/phrase you wrote down for "Light and Sight" on page 22. Does it still describe your experience?

As you implement the Sleepless Night Rules, you may notice a pivot. This may be a new mindset, a small shift toward peace, rest, comfort, and joy, or maybe some initial success or newfound confidence. If so, write down a new word or phrase that describes your pivot. If not, don't worry — just keep going! Change is slow work and often occurs as small steps in a new direction. But each one is worth celebrating!

If you are not seeing any change, bring your frustrations to God. Reflect on your most recent sleepless night and identify the rule you are having difficulty implementing.

_____

_____

_____

_____

_____

_____

_____

_____

_____

Remember Your Day

Take some time to journal about your day by responding to the prompts below or jotting down moments as they come to you.

What do you want to remember about this day?

_____

_____

_____

_____

_____

_____

_____

What do you want to forget?

_____

_____

_____

_____

_____

_____

_____

What else do you want to note about today?

_____

_____

_____

_____

_____

_____

_____

_____

_____

_____

_____

_____

_____

_____

_____

_____

_____

_____

_____

Rest Area

Whether you have had success already or are waiting to experience a change, commit to a consistent wake time and no naps for one week. Shade in a *Z* for each day you're successful!

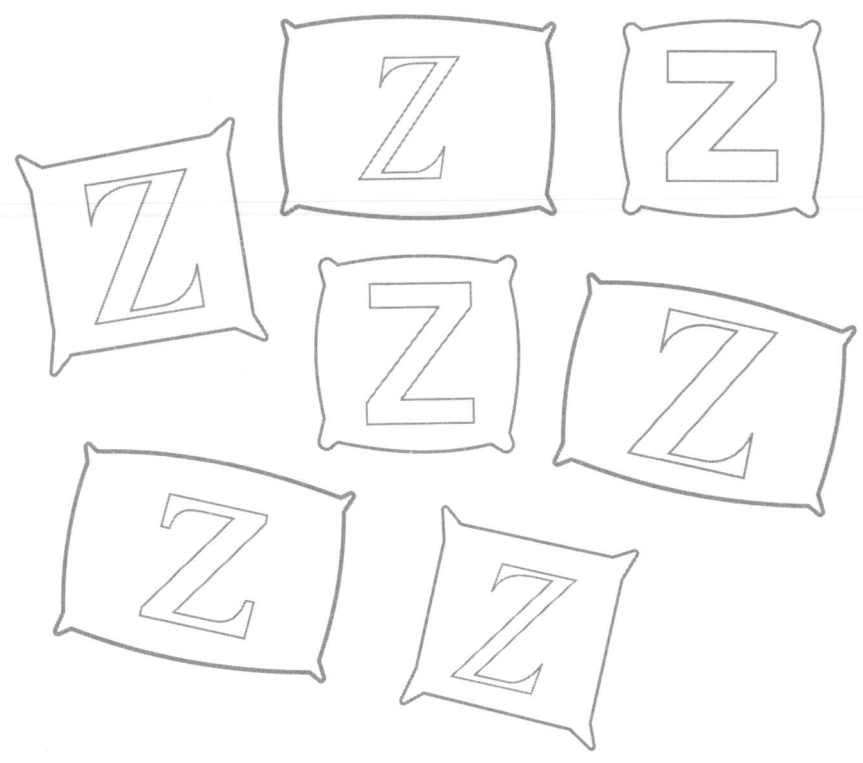

TRACKING YOUR
Sleep Journey

This week, estimate how long it takes to fall asleep (i.e., amount of time from initial lights out/head on the pillow to falling asleep).

NIGHT 1	
NIGHT 2	
NIGHT 3	
NIGHT 4	
NIGHT 5	
NIGHT 6	
NIGHT 7	

Insomnia is a glamorous
term for thoughts you
forgot to have in the day.

—ALAIN DE BOTTON

If you can't sleep, then
get up and do something
instead of lying there
worrying. It's the worry
that gets you, not the
lack of sleep.

—DALE CARNEGIE

Rise

Rise from bed if you cannot fall asleep.

The act of rising is critical to the sleepless night. In his book *Atomic Habits*, James Clear describes "decisive moments" as ones that "deliver an outsized impact … [that] set the options available to your future self."* When you recognize your sleeplessness, your choice of whether or not to get out of bed sets your options for the rest of the night. If you struggle with this step, it may be because you frequently think that sleep is "just around the corner." But staying in bed is not without consequence. Psychologically, rising out of bed is important because chronic tossing and turning creates a subconscious association between your bed and wakefulness. Theologically, you are a body and soul. What you do with your body, you also do to the soul. In light of this, rising becomes an embodied practice of trust and hope—a proactive rather than passive choice. When you stay in bed, insisting on sleep, you miss an opportunity to put your trust and hope into practice.

* James Clear, *Atomic Habits: Tiny Changes, Remarkable Results* (New York: Random House, 2018), 160–61.

Healthy Rising Habits

If you can't sleep, tossing and turning in bed, your problem is not failing to rise. Rather, it is that your system lacks sufficient motivation to rise. To paraphrase James Clear's "Four Laws of Behavior Change" in *Atomic Habits,* you need to make your getting out of bed more attractive.[*]

- **Pair it up!** Motivate yourself to get out of bed by pairing something you enjoy doing with getting out of bed. Write down some ideas below:

_____

_____

_____

_____

_____

_____

_____

_____

_____

_____

[*]   Clear, 53–54.

- **Carve out space.** Make the choice easier by identifying a space you can go to when you can't sleep.

- **Forgive one-offs.** One off night will not undo everything. But the most common break for a habit is the second night. The quicker you can get back to rising out of bed, the more likely you'll be to continue building the habit.

- **Remind yourself.** Sleep will not come more quickly just because you're lying down in bed. Tell yourself, "I'll come straight back to bed once I start to feel sleepy."

I'm sleepy when ...

☐ my eyes feel heavy.

☐ I nod off.

☐ I start yawning.

☐ I can't keep my eyes open.

☐

☐

☐

I'm Not Sleepy

Rather than focusing on how much time you should spend trying to fall asleep, focus on recognizing the moment you realize, *I'm not sleepy!* This might come as a thought or a feeling. Fill in the thought bubble with your signal that it's time to rise.

What Fires Together, Wires Together

Rising out of bed is important, because spending all night in your bed tossing and turning creates connections in your brain that tell you your bed is a place to be awake. The more you do in your bed (i.e., read, worry, scroll through your phone, toss and turn, do schoolwork, answer emails, etc.), the weaker the signal becomes that your bed is for sleeping.

Fill in the bed with any activities you do in bed. Then commit to making the bed a place for sleep by crossing out all the other options.

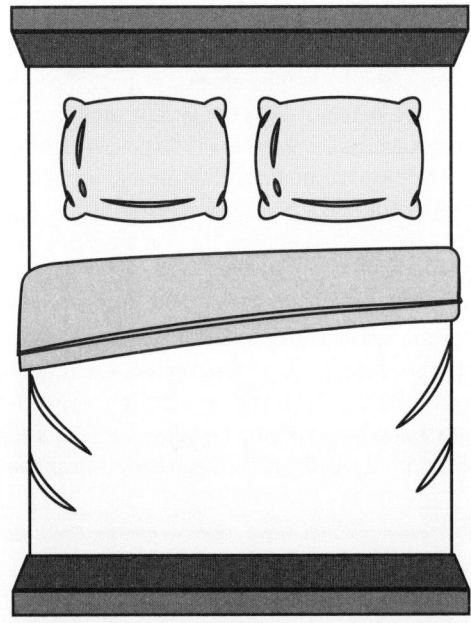

In Anguish

I am weary with my moaning;
　　　every night I flood my bed with tears;
　　　I drench my couch with my weeping.

　　　　　　　　　　　　　　　－Psalm 6:6, NRSVA

Illness can be isolating and painful. And too often, well-meaning Christians will spiritually bypass the discomfort in an effort to bring people hope. But the Psalms display over and over the importance of holding space for anguish.

The author of Psalm 6 pleaded for healing. Whether literal or metaphorical, this illness weighed on him every night and prompted him to cry, "Turn, Lord, and deliver me; save me because of your unfailing love" (verse 5, NIV). But instead of immediate deliverance, the author wept to the point that his "eye [wasted] away because of grief" (verse 7). And yet, by the end of the psalm, he declared that "the Lord has heard the sound of my weeping. The Lord has heard my supplication; the Lord accepts my prayer" (verses 8–9, NRSVA). This declaration is not "spiritual bypassing," or the use of spiritual or religious language and practices to circumvent suffering. Rather, it displays the tension of suffering against the existence of a good God. The psalm builds upon the idea that "the world as we have it is not the world as it should be or as God intended."[*]

The same can be said for your sleeplessness. Andrew Bishop writes that "deprivation or denial of sleep, whether imposed externally or generated physiologically, is always an affliction."[**] Your tossing and turning *is* an affliction, not to mention whatever else might be preventing

---

[*]　　Gerald Henry Wilson, *The NIV Application Commentary: Psalms Volume 1* (Grand Rapids, Mich.: Zondervan, 2002), 183.

[**]　　Andrew Bishop, *Theosomnia* (London and Philadelphia: Jessica Kingsley Publishers, 2018), 34.

you from falling asleep. The journey in this book gives space for acknowledging the depth of your current suffering without the pressure "to explain it away or find ways to interpret it positively."* May that truth bring you some measure of hope tonight.

Spend some time pouring out all your anguish to God.

_____

_____

_____

_____

_____

_____

_____

_____

_____

_____

_____

_____

_____

_____

_____

_____

*   Wilson, *The NIV Application Commentary: Psalms,* 184.

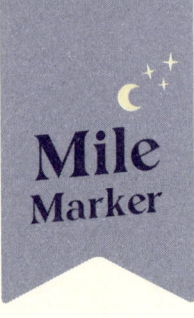

Mile Marker

Don't Give Up

Everyone will have moments on this journey when they will stagnate or regress. You may once again find yourself awake and dealing with the same problem—one step forward and three steps back. But the decisions you make when you are "three steps back" are where you can grow the most.

By consistently rising out of bed despite the same sleeplessness, you are becoming a certain kind of person. Rising is a "purposeful disruption of [your] 'automatic' thoughts, feelings, and actions" against the sleepless night.* It feels counterintuitive, but when you repeat this practice (especially on nights you *don't* want to do it), you're training yourself to become the kind of person who trusts God despite your circumstances.

Rising disrupts any illusion of control over sleep and creates an opportunity to humble yourself before God and trust that He loves you. Some nights you will get out of bed and God's love will be evident through sleepiness coming quickly. But other nights, God will use the sleepless night to invite you into deeper relationship with Him. Some nights you will experience God's love through more comfort, rest, peace, and joy despite the sleepless night. But if your hope is only for more or better sleep, then you might miss the potential for connection. Each night is a new opportunity. Even if you feel like you're failing, keep going. Get out of bed if you can't fall asleep, and see what God has in store for you.

---

* Dallas Willard, *The Divine Conspiracy: Rediscovering Our Hidden Life in God* (New York: HarperCollins, 1997), 322.

Go back to the "Hope" activity on page 23. Spend some time reflecting on what you were hoping for at the beginning of this journey and where you are now. Where is your hope tonight?

_____

_____

_____

_____

_____

_____

_____

_____

_____

_____

_____

_____

_____

_____

_____

_____

_____

_____

Sonnet 27

Weary with toil, I haste me to my bed,
The dear repose for limbs with travel tired;
But then begins a journey in my head,
To work my mind, when body's work's expired:
For then my thoughts, from far where I abide,
Intend a zealous pilgrimage to thee,
And keep my drooping eyelids open wide,
Looking on darkness which the blind do see:
Save that my soul's imaginary sight
Presents thy shadow to my sightless view,
Which, like a jewel hung in ghastly night,
Makes black night beauteous and her old face new.
Lo! Thus, by day my limbs, by night my mind,
For thee and for myself no quiet find.

—WILLIAM SHAKESPEARE

And Yet I Rise

Write a poem describing your sleeplessness and have each line end with
the phrase "and yet I rise."

An Embodied Hope

I rise before dawn and cry for help;
I have put my hope in your word.

—Psalm 119:147, **NIV**

Psalm 119 opens with "Blessed are those whose ways are blameless, who walk according to the law of the Lord" (**NIV**). The psalm continues to explore the law of the Lord not "as a strict set of rules and regulations but as a way of life or approach to being that brings one closer to God."* Try thinking in a similar way about getting out of bed when you can't fall asleep. Though rising from bed might feel counterintuitive when all you want to do is sleep, tossing and turning will get you nowhere. Sooner or later, you will be faced with the choice to stay put or get out of bed. And this choice is important for both the body and the soul.

Too often, we forget that what is done to the body is done to the soul. C. S. Lewis discusses this connection in *The Screwtape Letters,* saying that we assume "the bodily position makes no difference to [our] prayers"; while on the contrary, "whatever [our] bodies do affects [our] souls."** Rising forms your body and soul by acknowledging your creaturely limitations. It places your hope outside yourself and brings you closer to God. This doesn't mean that God hears your prayers better if you're in bed or out. Rather, your bodily position is a physical reminder that reorients your mind toward God. Rising relinquishes control and allows you to embody hope in your very being.

---

* Nancy deClaissé-Walford, *Psalms: Books 4–5,* Wisdom Commentary, vol. 22 (Collegeville, Minn.: Liturgical Press, 2020), 160.

** C. S. Lewis, *The Screwtape Letters, and Screwtape Proposes a Toast* (Québec: Pomodoro Books, 2020), 19.

Commit the opening verse to memory. When you recognize that you can't fall asleep, say this verse as a way of pivoting your attention toward God, and then rise out of bed.

What physical movements or stances make you feel more closely drawn to God? When have you experienced an "embodied hope?"

_____

_____

_____

_____

_____

_____

_____

_____

_____

_____

_____

_____

_____

_____

_____

_____

Embodied Connection

What you do with your body matters. Rising out of bed when you can't sleep moves your body and soul toward something else: hope instead of continual frustration, acceptance instead of despair. In addition, when you choose to connect with God, your body and soul move toward Someone else.

Within ancient Christian tradition, facing east during prayer was a communal practice to orient believers toward God. Since the sun rises in the east, it was thought, by some, to be the direction in which Jesus will return. Whether or not this is true, God is not contained to the east, nor does He need you to face the east in order to hear you better. Still, Augustine explained the eastward practice as being formative for the mind: "Our purpose is to impress upon our soul to turn to a more excellent nature, that is, to God, seeing that the body itself which is earthly, is turned to a more excellent body, that is, to a heavenly body."* In other words, this practice is to remind you of the connection between your body and spirit. What you do with your body reveals and forms your desires. So direct yourself toward the Light of the world.

Face east in your prayer time tonight and reflect on the promise that the sun will rise, this night will end, Christ will one day return, and your insomnia will be healed.

---

* Augustine of Hippo, *The Lord's Sermon on the Mount,* trans. John J. Jepson (Westminster, Md.: The Newman Press, 1948), 107.

Come to me, all you that are weary
and are carrying heavy burdens,
and I will give you rest.
            —Matthew 11:28, **NRSV**

I rise before dawn and cry for help;
    I hope in your words.
My eyes are awake before the watches
        of the night,
that I may meditate on your promise.
            —Psalm 119:147–148

Catch, Replace, Release

Are you believing any degenerative thoughts about your sleep? False or unhelpful thoughts like the ones listed below typically perpetuate insomnia. Use the columns below to catch your harmful thoughts and replace them with more helpful ones. Then give those negative thoughts to God.

DEGENERATIVE	RESTORATIVE
My sleep is out of control.	I can prepare to receive sleep as a gift.
I'll be a train wreck tomorrow if I don't get to sleep soon.	God has brought me through other days after a poor night's sleep.
I can't calm my mind enough to fall asleep.	I can take my thoughts captive and give them to God.
Insomnia is ruining my life. I have no energy to enjoy things or do what I want.	God can use my sleepless night to give me more rest, comfort, peace, and joy.
My sleep is beyond repair. I don't think anything will ever change that.	My sleep is part of the world's brokenness, but God can transform it.

A Prayer for Rising

Lord,
I'm tossing and turning.
Sleep has not come.
I know I should rise,
but what if sleep is just around the corner?
Give me courage to rise out of bed
and face this night.
Let my rising
remind me
that I put my hope in You.
You, O Lord, have brought me to this night,
and You will see me through it.

Write your own prayer to help you rise out of bed when you can't fall asleep.

_____

_____

_____

_____

_____

_____

_____

_____

_____

Remember Your Day

Take some time to journal about your day by responding to the prompts below or jotting down moments as they come to you.

When did you feel close to God today?

_____

_____

_____

_____

_____

_____

_____

When did God feel distant?

_____

_____

_____

_____

_____

_____

_____

What else do you want to note about today?

For the next week, commit to rising from bed when you can't fall asleep. Shade in an arrow for each night you're successful!

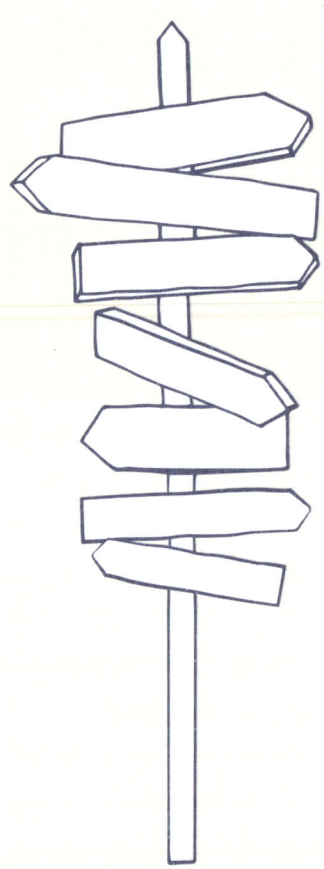

TRACKING YOUR
Sleep Journey

This week, track how many times you rise
out of bed during the night.

NIGHT 1	
NIGHT 2	
NIGHT 3	
NIGHT 4	
NIGHT 5	
NIGHT 6	
NIGHT 7	

Every hour of every day,
God is richly blessing us;
both when we sleep and
when we wake His mercy
waits upon us.

—CHARLES SPURGEON

Connect

Connect with God.

Connecting with God is at the heart of the Sleepless Night Rules. In this section, you will learn three ways to navigate sleeplessness from a Christian worldview—by remembering God's history, resting in the present, and watching the future.

Jesus once said, "Come to me, all you that are weary and are carrying heavy burdens, and I will give you rest" (Matthew 11:28, NRSV). As mentioned previously, you don't need eight hours of sleep to flourish. Sleep that is open to God and offered to God is transformative. God is the source of peace, rest, comfort, and joy in your sleepless night. Your task is to choose connection with Him so that you can find rest for your soul.

Presence over Productivity

Tremble, and do not sin;
Meditate in your heart upon your bed,
and be still. *Selah*

—Psalm 4:4, NASB

Do you ever think, *Well, if I can't sleep, I might as well be productive*? Sleep health professionals sometimes prescribe mundane tasks such as clearing clutter, folding clothes, or sorting through mail to fill one's sleepless time. While there isn't anything wrong with these suggestions, the biblical authors have a different vision. One that does not place a high value on usefulness and efficiency—both of which may cultivate a spirit of "anxious toil" (Psalm 127:2) within your heart—but instead directs people back toward a relationship with God.

In Psalm 4, the author addressed those who do not honor God and "love what is worthless and aim at deception" (verse 2, NASB1995). It seems some individuals within Israel "sought relief from their agricultural problems by appealing for deliverance to false gods."* The psalmist, on the other hand, knew that "the LORD hears when [he calls] to Him" (Psalm 4:3, NASB).

Even though we may not bow before physical idols, we still succumb to the same logic as those offering sacrifices to other gods. When sleep is out of reach, what you choose to do in the night reveals the desires of your heart. And for many of us, it is incredibly difficult to be unproductive. Can you connect with God while folding socks? Of course! These aren't

---

* Gerald Henry Wilson, *NIV Application Commentary: Psalms Volume 1* (Grand Rapids, Mich.: Zondervan, 2002), 154.

mutually exclusive. But character is revealed when plans go awry, and "what human beings do in their beds offers a telling picture of what they are doing with their lives: beds can gauge rest, sloth, pain, true residence, and the privacy and purity of the human heart."* When you rise out of bed and choose to be "unproductive" by being still and connecting with God, you are being countercultural. You are forming your heart away from someone who needs to make "good use of their time," and into someone who chooses to rest in God's presence and provision by being still in the present moment.

With what do you typically choose to fill your time when you can't sleep?

_____

_____

_____

_____

_____

_____

_____

_____

_____

_____

* *Dictionary of Biblical Imagery,* ed. Leland Ryken et al. (Downers Grove, Ill.: InterVarsity Press, 1998), 86.

Cross Out the List

Make a list of all the things you typically do or think you should do if you can't sleep. Then cross them out one by one and give them to God. (If you find yourself thinking about your to-do list, unpack it on pages 44–45).

✕ _____
✕ _____
✕ _____
✕ _____
✕ _____
✕ _____
✕ _____
✕ _____
✕ _____
✕ _____
✕ _____
✕ _____
✕ _____
✕ _____
✕ _____
✕ _____
✕ _____
✕ _____
✕ _____
✕ _____
✕ _____
✕ _____

Avoid the Algorithm

For many Christians today, social media and streaming platforms are by far the greatest distracter from connecting with God in their sleeplessness. Faceless algorithms are designed to keep our attention for as long as possible, and they are just as likely to suggest something shocking and inflammatory as they are relaxing and encouraging.

If over-connection to your phone is something you struggle with, consider trying these algorithm alternatives to help you get back to God and His gift of sleep.

- **Lock your phone.** Adjust the settings on your phone or download an app that limits your access overnight.

- **Keep your phone away from your bed.** If you use it as an alarm, buy an old-school alarm clock to use instead.

- **Delete social media apps from your phone.** If this feels too difficult, use a timer to help you limit your time on specific apps.

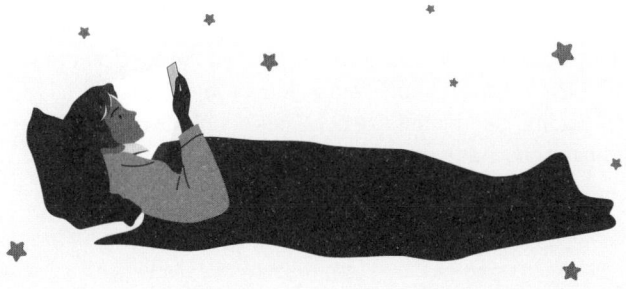

My Song in the Night

You have held my eyelids open;
I am so troubled that I cannot speak.
I have considered the days of old,
The years of long ago.
I will remember my song in the night;
I will meditate with my heart,
And my spirit ponders.

–Psalm 77:4–6, **NASB**

Barriers to good rest can feel overwhelming. The speaker in Psalm 77 is so troubled that it leaves him speechless and unable to sleep. But the psalm does not end with this focus on distress. Rather, the speaker turns to "the days of old" and remembers previous songs in the night. This choice to remember becomes a theme for the rest of the psalm and displays a path through the sleepless night.

When you remember who God is and what He has done, you're more able to turn away from despair and toward hope. Trouble does have a way of creating a nearsighted focus on current circumstances. It can be difficult to shift your perspective. But that is precisely how the Psalms reshape your thinking. Many psalms start by acknowledging the pain and trouble of current circumstances, but they soon turn to remembrance. This demonstrates how current sorrows facilitate the conditions for connection. It is not an attempt to erase your problems. Rather, it is a reminder that "the insurmountable becomes doable as we remember the God who in the past has worked miracles to help his people."[*]

---

* W. Dennis Tucker Jr. and Jamie A. Grant, *The NIV Application Commentary: Psalms Volume 2* (Grand Rapids, Mich.: Zondervan, 2018), 135.

How has God transformed the insurmountable into the doable in your life?

_____

_____

_____

_____

_____

_____

_____

_____

_____

_____

_____

_____

_____

_____

_____

_____

Explore More

Read Psalm 77:7–9 (NASB1995):

> Will the Lord reject forever?
> And will He never be favorable again?
> Has His lovingkindness ceased forever?
> Has His promise come to an end forever?
> Has God forgotten to be gracious,
> Or has He in anger withdrawn His compassion? *Selah*

The psalmist expressed his doubts as he questioned God, but these are not random questions. Rather, they are a window into the mind of the author.

Now read Exodus 34:6–7 (NASB1995):

> The LORD, the LORD God, compassionate and gracious,
> slow to anger, and abounding in lovingkindness and
> truth; who keeps lovingkindness for thousands, who
> forgives iniquity, transgression and sin.

These verses from Exodus mark the first time in the Old Testament that God describes His character. The revelation is so important that this group of verses is "one of the most quoted passages in the Bible."*

Now return to Psalm 77 and circle or highlight words that are also found in the passage from Exodus.

Whether the psalmist was reflecting on Exodus 34 explicitly or a song referencing it, the series of questions in Psalm 77 reveal that the author was meditating on the character of God and the tension between that and the psalmist's own circumstance.

---

*   "Visual Commentary: Exodus 34:6–7," Bible Project, June 30, 2020, https://bibleproject.com/explore/video/character-of-god-exodus..

The remainder of Psalm 77 unfolds as a reality check for the author. After recognizing the incongruence between God's character and the present situation, the psalmist then turned to God's history.

Read Psalm 77:10–20.

What moments from Israel's history are evident in the remainder of the psalm?

_____

_____

_____

_____

Who does the psalmist remember?

_____

_____

By remembering God's track record throughout the psalm, the psalmist moved beyond his current circumstance and saw the bigger picture of God's redemptive work with His people.

Though it might be hard right now to see God's redemptive work in your situation of sleeplessness, try to turn your thoughts of despair or frustration toward God's powerful character. And as you remember that God performed wondrous works throughout history, know that He can bring you rest, comfort, and joy in your sleeplessness.

Connect in the Mundane

As nourishing as time with God is, a nightly, mini-monastic spiritual retreat is not realistic for all of us. Demands from our day leave us with dishes to be done, laundry to be folded, and bills to be paid. On top of that, demands on our *night* may include caring for a family member, attending night school, juggling a second or third job, or cleaning up after a puppy. It is one thing to have difficulty being still due to a high value on productivity (see "Presence over Productivity" on pages 100–101), but it is another thing to find yourself in a season where you cannot retreat to any stillness in the night. So, invite God to bring the stillness to you.

How can you connect with God in the chaotic or mundane tasks that fill your sleepless night? Search for opportunities to shift your mind toward God. It can even be as small as taking a deep breath and calling upon His name.

_____

_____

_____

_____

_____

_____

_____

_____

_____

_____

Remember Your History

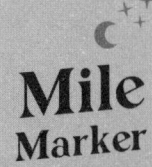

Reflect on your "Sleep History" from pages 14–15.
How has God moved in your life despite your sleep
problems? When have you experienced His mercy,
grace, patience, love, and truth in miraculous ways? How has He calmed
previous storms for you?

_____

_____

_____

_____

_____

_____

_____

_____

_____

_____

_____

_____

_____

_____

Gospel Meditation

Relationship with God happens when we share life with Him. One way we can build friendship with God is through the practice of gospel meditation. Dr. David G. Benner explains in *The Gift of Being Yourself,* "Gospel meditation provides an opportunity to enter specific moments in Jesus' life and thereby share his experience."[*]

Practice

- Find a quiet place and take a moment to "ask God to take the words of Scripture and, by the power of his Spirit, make them God's Word to you. Ask for the gift of a few moments of Spirit-guided imaginative encounter with Jesus."[**]

- Slowly read through the following passage at least twice.

- Allow yourself to enter the story and, "as if you were a spectator, observe the events as they unfold. Watch, listen and stay attentive to Christ. . . . And don't try to analyze the story or learn lessons from it. Just be present to Jesus and open to your own reactions."[***]

---

[*]   David G. Benner, *The Gift of Being Yourself: The Sacred Call to Self-Discovery* (Downers Grove, Ill.: InterVarsity Press, 2015), 37.

[**]   Benner, 37.

[***]   Benner, 38.

Jesus went out as usual to the Mount of Olives, and his disciples followed him. On reaching the place, he said to them, "Pray that you will not fall into temptation." He withdrew about a stone's throw beyond them, knelt down and prayed, "Father, if you are willing, take this cup from me; yet not my will, but yours be done." An angel from heaven appeared to him and strengthened him. And being in anguish, he prayed more earnestly, and his sweat was like drops of blood falling to the ground.

When he rose from prayer and went back to the disciples, he found them asleep, exhausted from sorrow. "Why are you sleeping?" he asked them. "Get up and pray so that you will not fall into temptation."

—Luke 22:39–46, **NIV**

Connecting in the Storm

And they came to Him and woke Him, saying, "Save us,
Lord; we are perishing!"

—Matthew 8:25, NASB

Have you ever lost hope in the middle of a challenging or stormy season
in your life? That is exactly how the disciples reacted in Matthew 8. The
winds were so strong, the waves were so great, and the boat was already
taking on so much water, that they couldn't imagine any future where they
would come out alive. But the answer to the storm was with them, sleeping
in the boat. The disciples woke Jesus and cried for help even as they
assumed they would perish. The Greek word for "perishing," *apollymetha,*
conveys a complete destruction (i.e., death is imminent).[*] The disciples
came to Jesus not in faith but out of desperation.

Your sleepless night may feel equally overwhelming. You're exhausted,
and life is not getting any easier. If anything, you are barely holding on, and
sinking seems imminent. You may find yourself stuck in the mindset that
nothing will change and that this storm will last forever. But acknowledging
your helplessness may be the catalyst you need to connect. Your situation
doesn't have to be perfect. You don't have to wait until things are calmer,
better, or easier. Let your current storm drive you to cry out and seek
connection with the only One who can calm it.

---

[*] Bible Hub, s.v. *apollymetha,* https://biblehub.com/greek/apollumetha_622.htm.

Reflect on your current storm and tell God what you are feeling. Don't sugarcoat it! Cry for help and wait for the peace that only God can bring.

_____

_____

_____

_____

_____

_____

_____

_____

_____

_____

_____

_____

_____

_____

_____

_____

_____

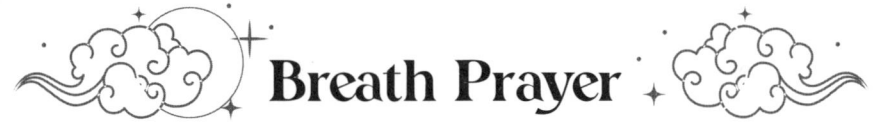

Breath Prayer

The most well-known breath prayer is the "Jesus Prayer," which echoes the words of a blind beggar named Bartimaeus. Jesus was leaving Jericho when Bartimaeus cried out the now famous words, "Jesus, Son of David, have mercy on me!" (Mark 10:47).

Practice

Find a place to be alone with God. Take some deep breaths and pray:

> Lord Jesus Christ,
> Son of God,
> have mercy on me.

A few variations in this practice include the following:

1. Saying each line while alternating inhaling and exhaling

2. Saying the whole prayer for the duration of one breath

3. Shortening the prayer to inhale while praying, "Christ," and exhale while praying "mercy"

If you become distracted, just continue. Try it for several minutes tonight and see if you can make it a habit this week.

The Serenity Prayer

God grant me the serenity
to accept the things I cannot change,
courage to change the things I can,
and wisdom to know the difference.

—Reinhold Niebuhr[*]

Use the lines below to write your own prayer or rewrite the prayer above.

_____

_____

_____

_____

_____

_____

_____

_____

_____

_____

---

[*]   Alcoholics Anonymous, "Origin of the Serenity Prayer: A Brief Summary," Service Material from the General Service Office, October 2, 2008, www.aa.org/origin-serenity-prayer-brief-summary.

Watching with Joy

Let the godly ones exult in glory;
Let them sing for joy on their beds.

−Psalm 149:5, NASB1995

If you've studied the Psalms, you may have noticed that lament is absent from the concluding chapters. The last five psalms all open with "Hallelujah," which means, "Praise the Lord!" These psalms focus on the promised future fulfillment of a messianic king who will conquer all evil. But this is not naïve optimism! Within its original context, the design to "end on a high note" comes after laments over both the destruction of Jerusalem and Israel's exile. But by meditating on the wisdom of the Psalms, the reader is able to make the journey from flooding one's bed with tears in Psalm 6 to singing for joy in Psalm 149. It just takes 143 chapters to come to fruition!

In the same way, years of sleeplessness might convince you there is no hope ahead. But the biblical narrative paints the picture of a King who will restore all creation. And for Christians, this restored reality is something we can experience now! Through Jesus's death and resurrection, we can sing for joy on our beds. We can hope in Christ as the source of our joy. We can look ahead to the restoration of all things through Jesus. And in the end, He will overturn the powers and principalities preventing good sleep in this world. The darkness of tonight cannot cancel out the hope ahead of you.

What is your initial reaction to this future joy? Spend some time reflecting on how real (or unreal) your hope in Christ feels right now.

_____

_____

_____

_____

_____

_____

_____

_____

_____

_____

_____

_____

_____

_____

_____

_____

_____

_____

Drawing New Creation

When it comes to sleeplessness, how can you move from present suffering to joy? Part of the transition is training your imagination to think differently about sleeplessness.

Imagine yourself in a city that "has no need of the sun or of the moon to shine on it, for the glory of God has illuminated it, and its lamp is the Lamb. The nations will walk by its light, and the kings of the earth will bring their glory into it. In the daytime (for there will be no night there) its gates will never be closed" (Revelation 21:23–25, NASB). A city that has no death, mourning, or pain. Where being awake means partnering with God and living forever refreshed and forever resting. Sleeplessness without suffering.

What comes to mind as you contemplate this picture of the new creation in Revelation?

Use the circle to draw what a redeemed, joyous sleeplessness in the new creation may look like.

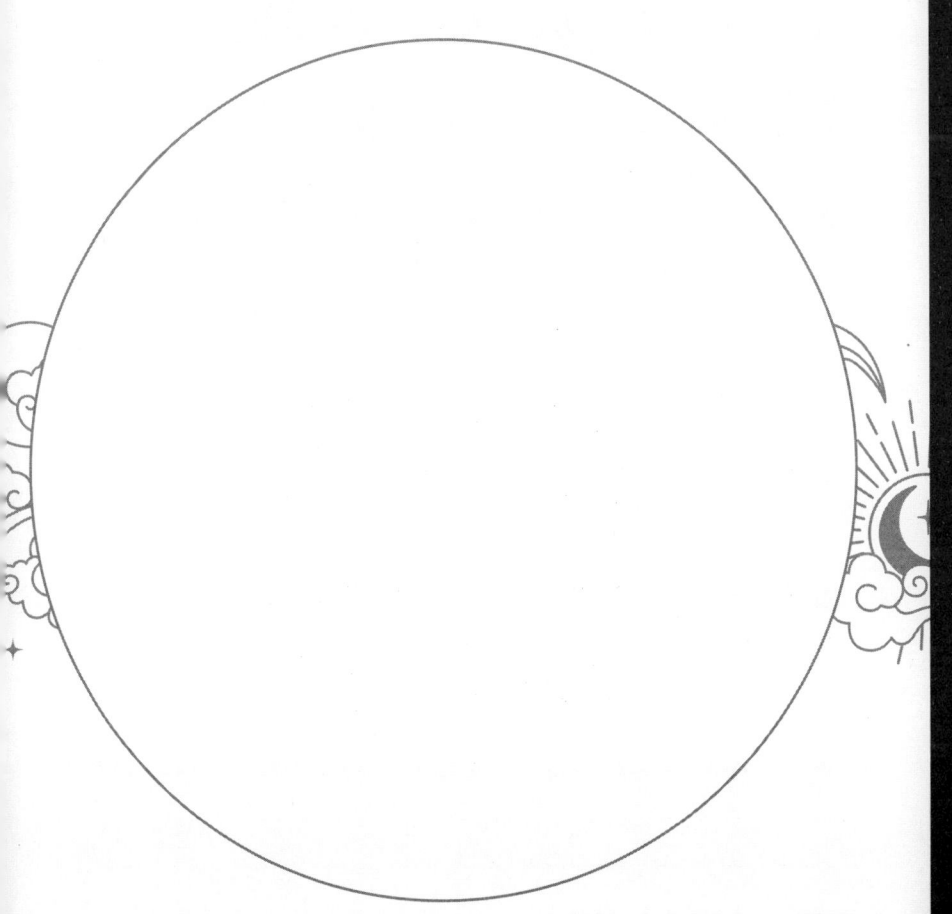

Remember Your Day

Take some time to journal about your day by responding to the prompts below or jotting down moments as they come to you.

When did you feel "not enough" today?

_____

_____

_____

_____

_____

_____

When did you experience a sense of triumph or accomplishment?

_____

_____

_____

_____

_____

_____

_____

What else do you want to note about today?

_____

_____

_____

_____

_____

_____

_____

_____

_____

_____

_____

_____

_____

_____

_____

_____

_____

_____

_____

Rest Area

Shade in a star for each sleepless night you find a way to connect with God.

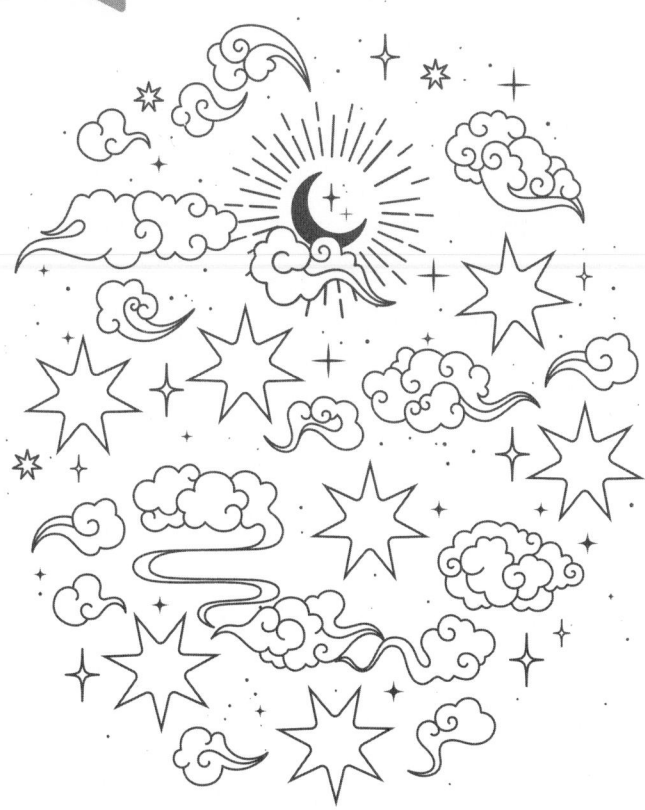

TRACKING YOUR
Sleep Journey

Track how you feel after connecting with God during the night.
Are you moving toward more peace, rest, comfort, and joy?

NIGHT 1	
NIGHT 1	
NIGHT 2	
NIGHT 3	
NIGHT 4	
NIGHT 5	
NIGHT 6	
NIGHT 7	

I lie awake;

I am like a lonely bird

on the housetop.

—PSALM 102:7, **NRSV**

Wait

Wait to feel sleepy.

Waiting to feel sleepy is trying. You might find yourself thinking, *I've gotta get some sleep,* or *It's been long enough,* or *It's time to lie down.* By its nature, this waiting is a test in patience. Nighttime provides a retreat from the responsibilities of the day and creates fertile ground for connection with God. For some, the silence and solitude of waiting in the night can be unsettling. Many will feel the impulse to do something. But as Nicetas of Remesiana once said, "With worldly occupations put aside and the attention undivided, the whole man, at night, stands in the divine presence."* It is here, without myriad distractions that fill your days, that God will meet with you and challenge you to grow in patience and trust.

*   Nicetas of Remesiana et al., *Writings; Writings; Commonitories; Grace and Free Will* (Washington, D.C.: Catholic University of America Press, 1949), 63.

Flip the Script

If you're anxious about being out of bed for too long or not feeling
sleepy, try flipping the script on your goal by focusing on staying awake
for just a little bit longer. Think of this as reverse psychology for your
sleep. By embracing the thing you're trying to avoid, you can reduce your
performance anxiety while paradoxically finding a pathway to feeling
sleepy again.

Embrace Your Fear with a New Script

Here's an example: "I'll stay awake for a little bit longer. I will sit here and
not feel sleepy. I will not yawn, and my eyes will not feel heavy." Repeat this
to yourself a few times and pause to see if you notice a difference. Feel
free to put a new spin on the script by writing your own version below:

_____

_____

_____

_____

_____

_____

_____

_____

_____

_____

Healthy Waiting Habits

If you're still waiting to feel sleepy, try:

- **Keeping your space dark.** Keep lights off or dimmed.

- **Maintaining a boring environment.** Strive for less mental engagement.

- **Remaining still.** Keep your activity level to a minimum (i.e., don't work up a sweat).

- **Avoiding food.** If you find yourself getting the munchies, let it pass. Eating is a signal for your brain to be awake.

- **Turning down the temperature.** Approximately 65–68 degrees Fahrenheit is a good range for a conducive sleep environment.[*]

---

[*]   Danielle Pacheco, "Best Temperature for Sleep," Sleep Foundation, March 7, 2024, www.sleepfoundation.org/bedroom-environment/best-temperature-for-sleep.

Feeling Impatient

If you're having difficulty staying out of bed long enough, use the space below to plan what you can do to counter impatience.

Instead of going back to bed earlier, I will _____

_____

_____

_____

_____

_____

_____

_____

_____

_____

_____

_____

_____

_____

_____

_____

_____

The Right Pizza Pan

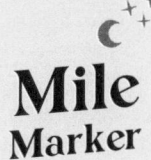

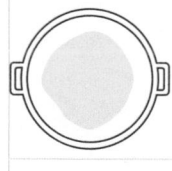

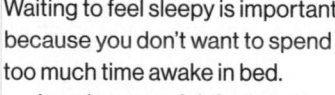

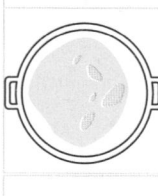

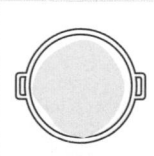

Waiting to feel sleepy is important because you don't want to spend too much time awake in bed.

Imagine your nightly sleep is a ball of pizza dough, and the time you spend in bed is your pizza pan. Since you have a limited amount of pizza dough, if you stretch it out too far, you're going to get rips. In other words, if you lie in bed beyond the amount of sleep your body needs, then you're going to wake up more in the night. So instead, try to make your pizza pan smaller by decreasing your time in bed to match your average nightly sleep plus around thirty minutes to give you time to fall asleep (e.g., for an average of five hours, you would decrease your time in bed to five hours and thirty minutes). Once you are falling asleep consistently within thirty minutes, increase the "size of your pizza pan" by ten minutes every few days. If you start having difficulty falling asleep, go back to your last successful amount of time in bed.

Write your average nightly sleep from page 30 in the pizza pan below.

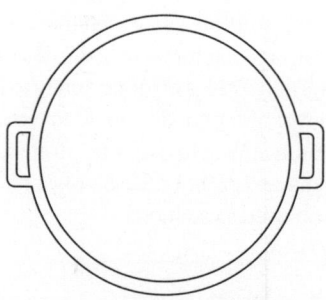

Building Patience

For I have learned to be content with whatever I have.
I know what it is to have little, and I know what it is
to have plenty. In any and all circumstances I have
learned the secret of being well-fed and of going
hungry, of having plenty and of being in need.

–Philippians 4:11–12, NRSVA

Any circumstance is an invitation to be present *in Christ.* In this passage, Paul thanked the Philippians for their support but also told them that he was content in any circumstance. The next verse reveals where he gets his ability to withstand the highs and lows: "Whatever I have, wherever I am, I can make it through anything in the One who makes me who I am" (verse 13, MSG). His contentment is developed not through receiving material comforts but through enduring various trials that bring about "perseverance; and perseverance, proven character; and proven character, hope" (Romans 5:3–4, NASB).

Similarly, waiting for sleep is a trial that can benefit your soul. You may have convinced yourself that coming back every night and waiting for sleep is crazy, because nothing seems to change. If your metric for change is getting eight hours of sleep, then you may have an argument. However, if waiting is part of training in patience, then your argument falls flat because patience is earned in waiting. Just like muscles become stronger when they are tested, so also your patience strengthens when you wait. Hope, joy, rest, and comfort are available to you, but you must consistently practice. Each night is an opportunity to be there *in Christ.* Repeatedly getting out of bed, choosing to direct your attention toward God, and accepting His invitation to connect is transformative. Seasons of sleeplessness will come and go, but consistently spending them in Christ builds the patience you need to continue.

Imagine Jesus waiting with you to feel sleepy. What would you do to pass the time?

_____

_____

_____

_____

_____

_____

_____

_____

_____

_____

_____

_____

_____

_____

_____

_____

_____

_____

_____

Waiting in Solidarity

> If you ever take your neighbor's cloak as a pledge, you are to return it to him before the sun sets, for that is his only covering; it is his cloak for his body. What else shall he sleep in? And it shall come about that when he cries out to Me, I will hear him, for I am gracious.
>
> –Exodus 22:26–27, NASB1995

God cares deeply about suffering—even suffering from disrupted sleep. The context of this passage from Exodus involves a poor man using his outer garment as collateral for some debt. While his thick cloak would be of little use during the heat of the day, it would be crucial for warmth at night. Anticipating this man's suffering, God commands the cloak's return so the man may sleep.

Likewise, God cares about your sleeplessness. And whether it is at the hands of people, systems, or circumstances, millions of people across the world will find themselves awake tonight—just like you. When we cry out to God, He is faithful to respond. He won't leave us alone or abandon us. Even if we've contributed to our sleeplessness by watching a thrilling show or drinking caffeine late in the day or taking a nap, God is not one to fold His arms and say, "I told you so." Suffering hurts His heart, and insomnia was never part of His design.

God's solution for this problem flows out of His gracious nature, which directs us toward right relationship with one another. In Deuteronomy, returning a neighbor's cloak is described as "righteousness for you before the Lord your God" (Deuteronomy 24:13, NASB). Reflecting on your suffering alongside that of fellow image-bearers brings your pain into community. This is not "spiritual bypassing." This is lament. Lament acknowledges that things are not as they are supposed to be, for you and for millions of others. In lament, you are saying, "Your pain is my pain." You join the cries of others asking our gracious God to intercede.

There is a certain peace in knowing you are not alone. So the next time sleep seems far off, cast your mind toward the sleeplessness of others in your community—the parents of a newborn, the newly widowed, the overworked, or the anxious.

Wait in solidarity with them. Cry out to God for wrongs to be made right. Wait, knowing that God will hear us, is gracious, and will send far more than cloaks for our bodies. He sent His Son, and He will do it again.

How does it feel to know you are not alone in your sleeplessness? What is your response when you reflect on your sleeplessness as part of a community?

_____

_____

_____

_____

_____

_____

_____

_____

_____

_____

_____

What's the Worst That Could Happen?

Write down the worst thing that could happen because you cannot sleep (e.g., I'll lose my job, I'll get in a car crash, etc.). This should be something you think of frequently when you're trying to fall asleep. After you identify a few thoughts, try to gauge how *certain* you feel these things will happen in the moment. Picture yourself lying in bed and thinking these thoughts. On a scale of 0 to 100 percent, how likely do you think it is that the worst thing will actually happen the next day?

WORST THAT COULD HAPPEN	HOW LIKELY I EXPECT IT TO HAPPEN
I lose my job	65%

WORST THAT COULD HAPPEN	HOW LIKELY I EXPECT IT TO HAPPEN

Now fill in the blanks to estimate how many sleepless nights you have experienced in your entire life.

I have trouble with my sleep _____ (nights per week) x 52 = _____ x _____ (number of years with sleep problems) = _____ (total number of sleepless nights)

Example: Poor sleep 4 nights/week for 10 years is 4 x 52 = 208 x 10 = 2,080 sleepless nights!

Now use that total number of sleepless nights to test your fear against reality. Let's say you're afraid of losing your job because you lost your job once after a poor night's sleep. To find the likelihood of that happening again, divide the times your fear has actually occurred by your total number of sleepless nights.

Example: Lost my job 1 time ÷ 2,080 total sleepless nights = 0.0004

To see this as a percentage, multiply by a hundred:
0.0004 x 100 = 0.04%,
which is the frequency your fear has actually occurred.

Finally, let's find out how many times your fear *should* have happened based on how you worry about it at night. If most nights you feel like you are 65 percent sure you will lose your job because of poor sleep, then you would divide the percentage by 100 and then multiply that by your total number of previous sleepless nights.

Example: I'm 65 percent sure I'll lose my job ÷ 100 = 0.65. Then 0.65 x 2,080 (total sleepless nights) = 1,352 times you should have lost your job based on how likely you expect it to happen while trying to fall asleep.

TIMES THE FEAR HAS ACTUALLY OCCURRED	FREQUENCY THE FEAR HAS ACTUALLY OCCURRED	FREQUENCY I EXPECT THE FEAR TO HAPPEN	TIMES THE FEAR SHOULD HAVE HAPPENED
1	0.04%	65%	1,352

TIMES THE FEAR HAS ACTUALLY OCCURRED	FREQUENCY THE FEAR HAS ACTUALLY OCCURRED	FREQUENCY I EXPECT THE FEAR TO HAPPEN	TIMES THE FEAR SHOULD HAVE HAPPENED

As you can see, the things you are afraid will happen because you can't sleep are often actually less than 1 percent. Returning to this formula can help you have more peace when you start worrying about these fears in the future.

Watching While Waiting

> Therefore let us not sleep, as others do, but let us watch and be sober.
>
> —1 Thessalonians 5:6, NKJV

Most theologians don't take Paul literally in this verse, since Paul was using sleep to describe individuals who are not ready for the "Day of the Lord" (i.e., Jesus's return). But what exactly does it mean to *watch*?

In the original Greek, *grēgoreō* is used by Jesus in the Gospels to convey a cautious, strict attention for when Jesus, the master of the house, will return (see Matthew 24:42; 25:13; Mark 13:35). But suffering makes watching difficult. It is hard to hold on to the joy of Jesus's return when life is filled with so much hurt. But by turning your mind toward Jesus's return, you are planting yourself firmly in between what Jesus has already done and the joy that is ahead of you.

The life, death, and resurrection of Jesus started the process of bringing heaven down to earth. Now all of creation lives in this in-between of the "here and not yet." God is near *and* real suffering continues. But Christians have an expectant hope. Watching and waiting in the night leans into the tension of Jesus's return and our present suffering. The Psalms sum it up beautifully: "My soul waits in hope for the Lord more than the watchmen for the morning; yes, more than the watchmen for the morning" (Psalm 130:6, NASB). Just as there is joy in the anticipation of a sunrise, so there is joy in anticipation of Jesus's return. But we miss that joy if we don't watch for it.

As you wait for sleep to fall, set your mind on Christ's return. Ask God to let the joy of this truth sink deeper into your heart. Let it take root in such a way that your confidence in Christ's return is as sure as the dawn.

What is your response to the idea that Jesus's return is as sure as the sun rising tomorrow?

_____

_____

_____

_____

_____

_____

_____

_____

_____

_____

_____

_____

_____

_____

_____

_____

_____

_____

Practicing Gratitude

Good things come to those who wait, even if it doesn't feel like it in the waiting. But sometimes it's not until you look back that you realize you're thankful God didn't give something to you on your timeline. Write three things you are grateful for, with at least one of them being something that was worth the wait.

1. _____

2. _____

3. _____

Noticing the Good

One way to move toward more peace and comfort in your night is to be open to experiencing God's goodness. Consider how James tells us that "every generous act of giving, with every perfect gift, is from above, coming down from the Father of lights" (James 1:17, NRSVA). God moves in the world by the good you experience and participate in throughout the course of your day. It is not some amorphous thing in the future. God's goodness is the surprise of the present that cuts through difficult circumstances and leaves you with a sense of wonder, joy, and presence.

What good have you experienced or participated in recently?

_____

_____

_____

_____

_____

What was the last thing to make you laugh or smile?

_____

_____

_____

_____

_____

Waiting Through Compline

One way we can discover rest in our nights of sleeplessness is by turning our thoughts toward others—specifically those closest to us. This practice is not meant to send you on a guilt trip or to minimize what you are experiencing. Rather, it is meant to shift your perspective outward. The practice of Compline (a form of liturgical prayer recited at night) helps us think beyond our own sleeplessness and provides a framework to join in solidarity with the sleeplessness of others.

Compline Prayer*

Write down the names of those who come to mind for the statements below and then spend time praying for each of them.

Keep watch, dear Lord, with those who:

Work: _____

Watch: _____

Weep: _____

Tend the sick: _____

Give rest to the weary: _____

Bless the dying: _____

Soothe the suffering: _____

Pity the afflicted: _____

Shield the joyous: _____

---

*   *Book of Common Prayer* (New York: Church Hymnal Corporation), 134, www.bcponline.org.

Silence and Solitude

John Ortberg describes the practice of silence and solitude as "forcing you to live with your consciousness without any distractions."* Keeping that in mind, sit in silence for five minutes without anything to distract you and write down whatever thoughts come to your mind. If you are not sleepy at the end of the five minutes, spend some time talking to God about your experience.

_____

_____

_____

_____

_____

_____

_____

_____

_____

_____

_____

_____

_____

*   John Ortberg, interview with John Mark Comer and Bethany Allen, "Solitude 02: The Quiet Place with John Ortberg," *Rule of Life,* Practicing the Way, podcast audio, September 21, 2023, https://podcasts.apple.com/us/podcast/solitude-02-the-quiet-place-with-john-ortberg/id1646299048?i=1000628671015.

Distracting Thoughts

Waiting is often self-revelatory, uncovering thoughts or worries that might remain buried when we're constantly on the go. Early Christians "identified eight types of thoughts, which distracted them from following Jesus, becoming more like him, and living out a set of virtues."[*]

Sometimes the sleepless night reveals the one spirit that "assails you unceasingly during your standing, walking, sitting, movement, rising, prayer, and sleep."[**]

Use the chart to assess whether your thoughts in the night fit under a spiritual vice. Then take that thought captive and give it to the Lord.

SPIRITUAL VICE[***]	DISTRACTING THOUGHT
Envy—"irrational sadness over another's good fortune"	
Anger—reaction to a perceived injustice	
Pride—"disordered self-love or irrational desire for self-exaltation"	

---

[*]   Joshua J. Knabb, *Christian Meditation in Clinical Practice: A Four-Step Model and Workbook for Therapists and Clients* (Downers Grove, Ill.: InterVarsity Press, 2021), 166.

[**]   John Climacus, *The Ladder of Divine Ascent* (Mahwah, N.J.: Paulist Press, 1982), 190.

[***]   Brant Pitre, *Introduction to the Spiritual Life: Walking the Path of Prayer with Jesus* (New York: Image, 2021).

SPIRITUAL VICE	DISTRACTING THOUGHT
Lust—"disordered desire for sexual pleasure"	
Gluttony—"disordered or immoderate desire for pleasure of food or drink"	
Acedia—disordered inclination to "apathetic inaction or distracted and ceaseless busyness"**	
Greed—an "irrational or immoderate desire to acquire money or possessions"	
Sorrow—an "irrational response to evil, suffering, or loss"***	

* Brant Pitre, *Introduction to the Spiritual Life: Walking the Path of Prayer with Jesus* (New York: Image, 2021).

** James McMartin, "Sleep, Sloth, and Sanctification," *Journal of Spiritual Formation and Soul Care* 6, no. 2 (2013): 268.

*** *In Introduction to the Spiritual Life,* Brant Pitre contrasts this with "godly sorrow," which is a "reasonable response to evil, suffering, or loss. . . . It does not exaggerate but faces evil or loss directly and realistically. [It] leads to repentance, trust in God, and eternal life" (pages 185–186).

Write a Letter

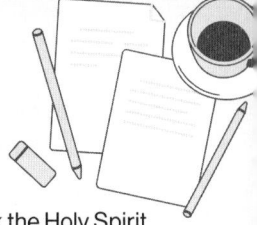

Spend the sleepless part of your night writing a letter. Ask the Holy Spirit to bring someone to mind. It could be a friend, your mailman, a family member, or anyone else. Whether you choose to send it is up to you.

_____

_____

_____

_____

_____

_____

_____

_____

_____

_____

_____

_____

Remember Your Day

Take some time to journal about your day by responding to the prompts below or jotting down moments as they come to you.

How did you fill your time whenever you had to wait?

_____

_____

_____

_____

_____

_____

Where does your mind go when you are waiting in line, at your computer, or in traffic?

_____

_____

_____

_____

_____

_____

_____

What else do you want to note about today?

_____

_____

_____

_____

_____

_____

_____

_____

_____

_____

_____

_____

_____

_____

_____

_____

_____

_____

_____

_____

Rest Area

For the next week, commit to staying out of bed until you feel sleepy. Shade in a yield sign for each night you're successful!

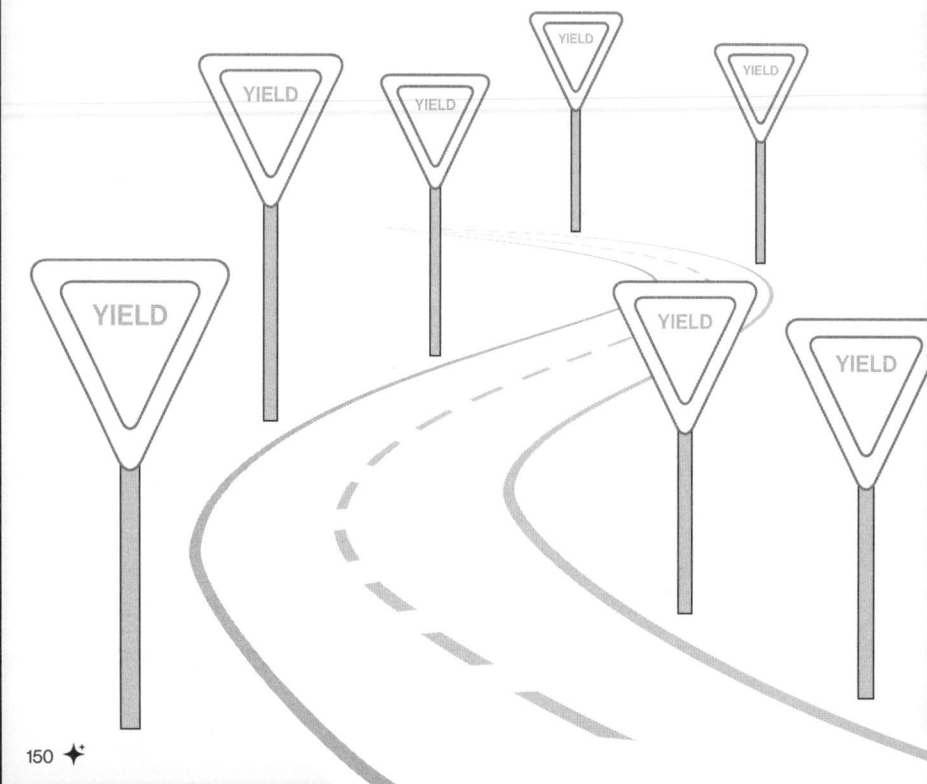

TRACKING YOUR
Sleep Journey

Track how long you are waiting to feel sleepy each night.

NIGHT 1	
NIGHT 2	
NIGHT 3	
NIGHT 4	
NIGHT 5	
NIGHT 6	
NIGHT 7	

I'm so good at sleeping that I can do it with my eyes closed.

—ANONYMOUS

Sometimes I lie awake at night, and I ask, "Where have I gone wrong?" Then a voice says to me, "This is going to take more than one night."

—CHARLES SCHULZ,
CHARLIE BROWN IN *PEANUTS**

---

* Stephen J. Lind, *A Charlie Brown Religion: Exploring the Spiritual Life and Work of Charles M. Schulz* (Jackson, Miss.: University Press of Mississippi, 2015), 124.

Repeat

Lie down and repeat rules
2 and 3 if you cannot fall asleep.

Repetition is the key to learning, but doing something over and over again doesn't necessarily make it any easier. Repeating the Sleepless Night Rules can often feel pointless. But consistency is key. Unfortunately, many people give up right at the critical moment when they need to continue. This is not to say you should ignore how you're feeling. Rather, it is a reminder that the night is always darkest before the dawn. Know that no matter how dark the night is tonight: "The steadfast love of the Lord never ceases; his mercies never come to an end; they are new every morning; great is [His] faithfulness" (Lamentations 3:22–23).

Grasp Gratitude

Poor mental health creates a chasm between you and joy. If you are in a difficult season, it is important to hold tightly on to gratitude—as well as to find support from a mental health professional and your community.

Use the following gratitude statements as proclamations of joy you can declare over yourself when you're feeling hopeless. I've provided two for you. Fill in the third with something you are grateful for—even if it's small.

1. I'm alive. Life is hard and painful, but it is also a gift.

2. I am completely known and loved by God. I am not loved for my potential or progress. I am known and loved for being me.

3. _____

Phone a Friend

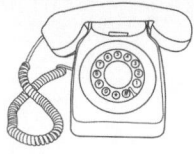

Sometimes we just need to know someone is there for us. Write down the names of three people who can encourage you and help keep you accountable as you continue your journey this week.

_____

_____

_____

Turned Toward Good

So the LORD God caused a deep sleep to fall upon the man, and he slept; then He took one of his ribs and closed up the flesh at that place.

—Genesis 2:21, NASB

Now when the sun was going down, a deep sleep fell upon Abram; and behold, terror and great darkness fell upon him.

—Genesis 15:12, NASB

The phrase "falling asleep" seems to accurately capture the elusiveness of sleep. By its nature, sleep is entered indirectly. You lie down and, in a way, pretend to sleep before it actually starts.

In the biblical narrative, sleep often comes within a sequence of blessing. God recognized both Adam's and Abram's loneliness and used sleep to bring about flourishing. Adam woke to meet Eve, and Abram witnessed God's promise for descendants. Adam's loneliness was transformed into a relationship. Abram's loneliness was transformed into a family that would bless all families. Sleep is a channel through which God brings about blessing.

But notice that Abram's sleep was overshadowed by terror, darkness, and oppression. Though sin had not yet entered the world at the time of Adam's sleep, Abram could not escape it—and neither can we. Sin impacts all of creation. Sleepless nights will repeat and repeat. But God can turn our sleeplessness into good. He did that with King Ahasuerus, whose sleeplessness led to the discovery of Mordecai's loyalty (see Esther 6:1–3). And He did that with an imprisoned Paul and Silas, whose prayers and singing at midnight preceded an earthquake that opened every prison door and broke every prisoner's chains (see Acts 16:22–29).

He also did it with the disciples, who, after spending an entire night trying to row across the sea, got to witness Jesus calming the wind (see Mark 6:45–52).

As you reflect on these stories, remember that the same God is watching over your sleep, and every night is an opportunity to think openly and flexibly about your sleep. Tonight, take comfort that the gift of sleep may fall on you quickly. But if it doesn't, then your sleeplessness is "infinitely overflowing with possibilities for grace and goodness."[*] God can turn both deep sleep and sleeplessness toward good.

Reflect on God bending your sleeplessness away from darkness, terror, and oppression and toward His good. Journal your response below.

_____

_____

_____

_____

_____

_____

_____

_____

---

[*]   Sheridan Hough, "First Movement: The *Aduton* of Selfhood," *Kierkegaard's Dancing Tax Collector: Faith, Finitude, and Silence* (Oxford: Oxford Academic, 2015; online ed. 2015), 29.

Redraw Your
Sleepless Night

Use the circle to draw what your nights look like
after implementing the Sleepless Night Rules.

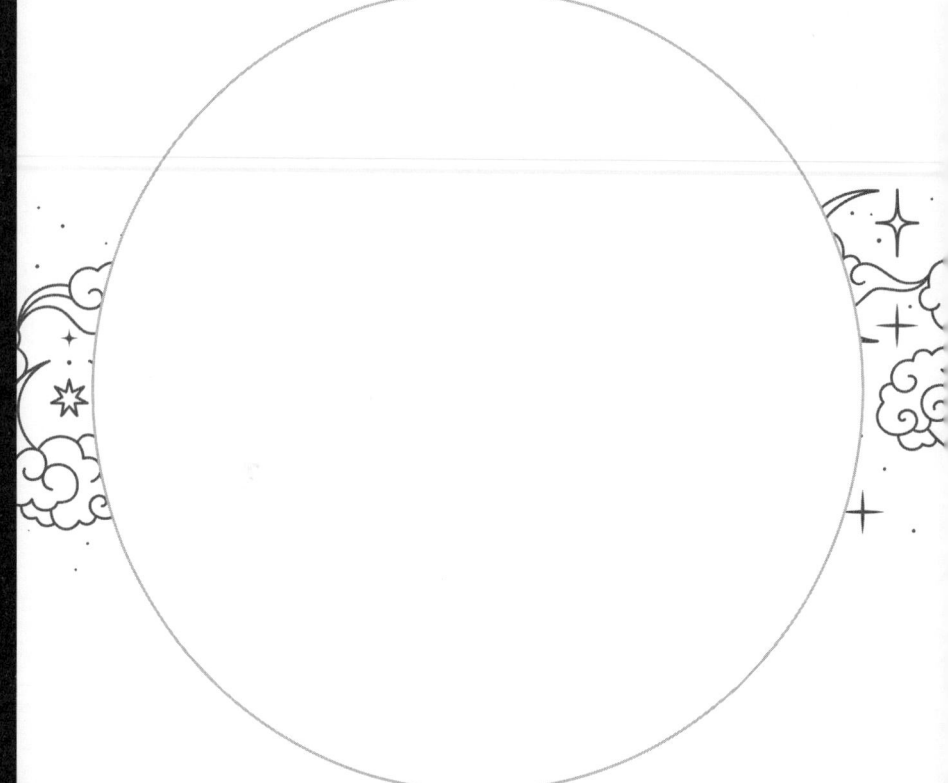

Now compare this circle with your previous drawings on pages 50–51.
Use the space below to reflect on the similarities and differences.

_____

_____

_____

_____

_____

_____

_____

_____

_____

_____

_____

_____

_____

_____

_____

_____

_____

_____

Small Bites

One of the biggest barriers to progress is biting off more than you can chew. We often set ambitious goals that are just out of reach and then become discouraged when we fail to accomplish them. So instead, let's focus on smaller bites.

Pick one of the Sleepless Night Rules. In the space below, break the rule down into small "bites" or steps. For instance, if you're going to cease before bed, ask yourself, "What do I need to do *before* bedtime to be ready to cease?"

Sleepless Night Rule: _____

- _____

- _____

- _____

- _____

- _____

Save Your Sleep Pressure

Consistency can be a challenge. But if you can at least wake up at the same time each day and avoid taking naps, you're off to a good start.

If you're still struggling, think of your sleep as a bank. You will likely have several rough nights at the beginning. But if you wake up consistently at the same time each morning, you will have more sleep pressure to help you fall asleep the next night. Each day you wake up at the same time—regardless of how good or bad the night before was—you are depositing any leftover sleep pressure into your "account." After a few days of doing that, you will have a balance to "cash in" and should notice it's a little easier to fall asleep.

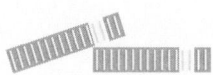
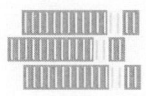

Sleepy vs. Fatigued

If implementing the rules results in no change for your daytime sleepiness, make sure you're noting the difference between feeling sleepy and feeling fatigued. If most of your symptoms fall in the fatigue category, consider talking with your doctor to explore your symptoms further.

Circle/highlight whatever best describes your sleepiness during the day.

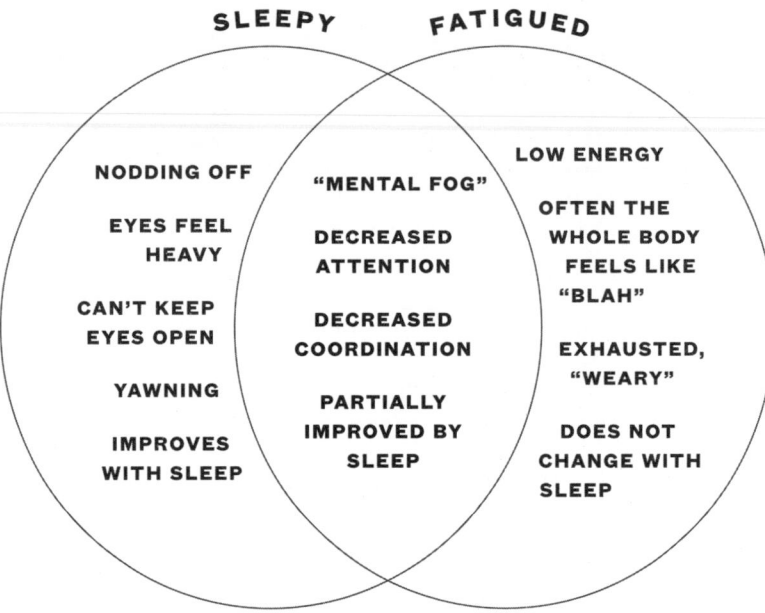

SLEEPY　　FATIGUED

NODDING OFF

EYES FEEL HEAVY

CAN'T KEEP EYES OPEN

YAWNING

IMPROVES WITH SLEEP

"MENTAL FOG"

DECREASED ATTENTION

DECREASED COORDINATION

PARTIALLY IMPROVED BY SLEEP

LOW ENERGY

OFTEN THE WHOLE BODY FEELS LIKE "BLAH"

EXHAUSTED, "WEARY"

DOES NOT CHANGE WITH SLEEP

Why Did I Do That?

When you're lying awake in bed, do you ever find yourself thinking about embarrassing things you did when you were younger? As your mind focuses on the negative outcome, you might struggle to remember that "little you" was doing the best he or she could for that age and under those circumstances. If you can, try to give your past self grace.

Use the space below to write down any embarrassing moments you tend to fixate on. Then ask God to bring to mind one or two positive moments from that time period and write those down as well.

_____

_____

_____

_____

_____

_____

_____

_____

_____

_____

_____

_____

_____

His Love Endures

> [W]ho made the great lights,
>> for his steadfast love endures for ever;
> the sun to rule over the day,
>> for his steadfast love endures for ever;
> the moon and stars to rule over the night,
>> for his steadfast love endures for ever.

—Psalm 136:7–9, NRSVA

Psalm 136 comes after a section of the Psalms called "the Songs of Ascents," which the Israelites would recite on pilgrimages to Jerusalem when observing holidays. Once they arrived in the city, this psalm would become a call to worship and "a truncated recitation of Israel's history."* The structure of the psalm remembers God as creator, deliverer, and sustainer. It also suggests a call and response format in which the priest "confesses the work of God and the people confess the faithfulness of God" with the repeated phrase "for his steadfast love endures forever" (twenty-six times to be exact).**

The Hebrew word for "steadfast love" is *hesed,* a notoriously difficult word for translators. It conveys a committed, trustworthy, and kind love. A love that speaks to the character of God. In this psalm, we can see *hesed* in the fact that God's deliverance and provision was not due to Israel's obedience, but rather due to God's own goodness.

In the same way, verses 7–9 of this psalm can serve as a reminder of God's *hesed* for *you* and of the truth that the night does not separate you from His love. When you've gotten out of bed two times already but still

---

* W. Dennis Tucker Jr. and Jamie A. Grant, *The NIV Application Commentary: Psalms Volume 2* (Grand Rapids, Mich.: Zondervan, 2018), 879.

** Tucker and Grant, 889.

can't sleep, remember that God is with you. When you have nights when you want to quit, remember that God's love never quits. And when your sleep journey feels endless, remember that God's transforming work in you is not finished yet. The God who created the heavenly lights is the same God who will deliver and sustain you in this night—for His steadfast love endures forever.

Reflect on God's trustworthy, committed, kind love. It is the same yesterday, tonight, and tomorrow.

_____

_____

_____

_____

_____

_____

_____

_____

_____

_____

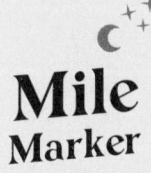

Mile
Marker

Reframe Your History

Write down some moments from your sleep journey, but this time add the phrase "His love endures forever" after each line. You could pick moments from your history (see pages 14–15 or 163), something you were grateful for (see pages 27, 42, 66, 140, or 154), or some other activity that stood out to you.

_____

_____

_____

_____

_____

_____

_____

_____

_____

_____

_____

_____

_____

A Prayer for Repeating

God,
I feel stuck.
I'm doing the same thing
over and over
but nothing changes.
I feel like giving up.
But Your love never quits.
You are gracious,
compassionate, slow to anger,
and abounding in steadfast love.

If I stopped trying for a thousand
    nights
You would still be there,
because You are unchanging.

So give me strength to follow You
    this night,
and every other night—
over and over.
Help me do the same thing,
by staying stuck on You.

Write your own prayer below.

_____

_____

_____

_____

_____

_____

_____

_____

_____

_____

_____

_____

_____

_____

_____

Geoffrey of Peronne

In *Introduction to the Devout Life,* Francis de Sales tells the story of Geoffrey of Peronne, who joined a monastery and found himself "in a state of dryness, and being deprived of consolation and overwhelmed with interior darkness." It seems that after taking his vows, Geoffrey was having second thoughts about everything he was giving up—his friends, family, and riches.

One of his friends in the monastery noticed a change and asked why he was so sad.

"Ah! My brother, I shall never be joyful again."

In his sorrow, Geoffrey laid his head on a stone and fell asleep. But after a little while, he rose from his sleep refreshed. It was such a change that his friend couldn't help but poke fun at Geoffrey's previous statement of never being joyful again.

Geoffrey answered, "If I told you a short while ago that I should never be joyful again, now I assure you that I shall never again be sad."[*]

As Geoffrey discovered, sometimes a short nap is precisely what we need to change our perspective. If you are struggling with resisting naps, allow yourself a short nap, limiting it to ten or fifteen minutes.

---

[*] Francis de Sales, *Introduction to the Devout Life,* trans. Allan Ross (London: Burns Oates and Washbourne, 1924), 278.

Draw yourself as Geoffrey, laying your head down to rest.

Rest Area

Commit to practicing all the rules every night for one week. Shade in an arrow for each night you're successful!

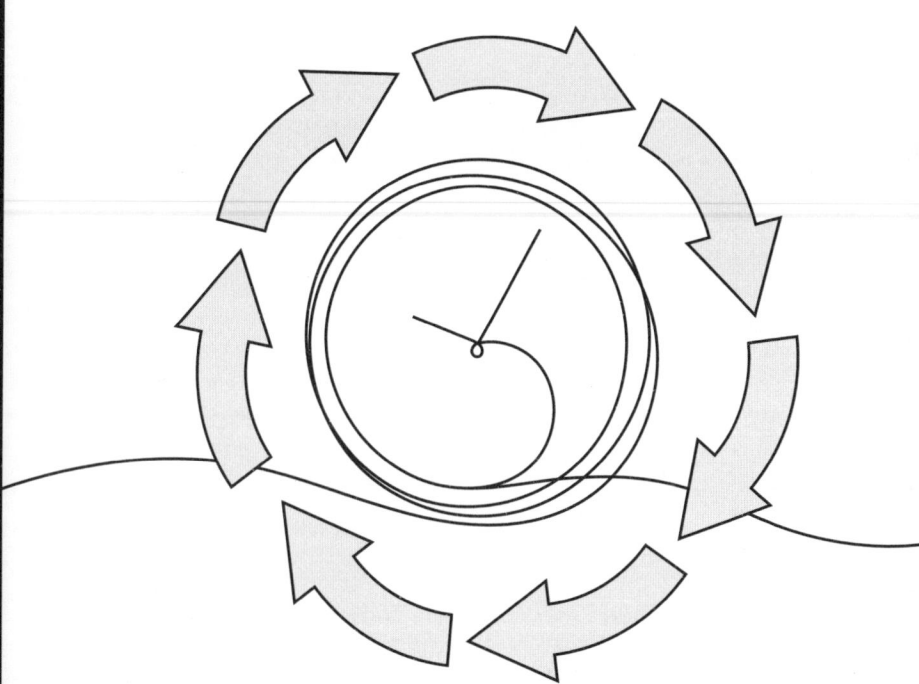

TRACKING YOUR
Sleep Journey

Estimate how much total sleep you're getting each night.

NIGHT 1	
NIGHT 2	
NIGHT 3	
NIGHT 4	
NIGHT 5	
NIGHT 6	
NIGHT 7	

The Journey Ahead

The sleepless night is a long and winding journey with highs and lows. Progress and regress. But with each trial comes the opportunity for *theosomnia*. When your sleep is offered to God, you discover a different way through the night. You don't need eight hours of sleep to flourish. You need God. The sleepless night will bring you back to that need again and again, and God is with you in it. Every season of sleeplessness is an opportunity to move toward Jesus's trusting posture of sleeping in the boat and watching on the mountainside. Celebrate each step toward peace, comfort, rest, and joy as you move closer to the promise of sleeplessness in new creation. No night. No suffering. Forever refreshed. Only light and eternal joy with God.

Index

Acknowledgments

I'm first and foremost grateful to God for this book. He put a passion in my heart and made a way when I thought it would never happen. Thanks to Great-grandma Thompson (who introduced me to books), Granddaddy (who never said no to buying me books), and my first pen pal, Grandpa Ralph, for planting a love of reading and writing in me. To Mom and Dad, for helping that love grow and always supporting me, encouraging me, and pushing me when I thought too little of myself. To Sydney, for your constant support and patience while listening to far too many diatribes on homeostatic regulation. To Oliver, for teaching me about sleepless nights, asking profound questions at bedtime, and being genuinely excited about all that I do.

To Jeff and my OG "How to Write a Book" Retreat crew: Y'all helped me believe I was a writer and gave me the courage that led me to write this book. Jordan, there is a direct line between your podcast and this book. I'm indebted to your enthusiastic support. To my agent Kristy: I was in way over my head and your support was a game changer. To Ink & Willow and all the staff at WaterBrook & Multnomah, thank you for taking a chance on me! Leslie, you have been so gracious with your feedback. Your edits elevated my writing to new heights. Finally, to all the patients and families I've had the honor of accompanying through sleepless nights: You have been, and always will be, my best teachers. This book would not exist without you.

About the Author

Benjamin Long is a sleep medicine physician with dual board certification in sleep medicine and pediatrics. He is an assistant professor of pediatrics with expertise in sleep disorders for all ages. As a seminary student, Ben enjoys writing at the intersection of sleep medicine and Christian theology. He lives with his wife and son in San Antonio, Texas.

01 14

√